Criminal Profiling

Criminal Profiling

Principles and Practice

Richard N. Kocsis, PhD
Forensic Psychologist

Foreword by

George B. Palermo, MD, MScCrim
Clinical Professor of Psychiatry and Neurology, Medical College of Wisconsin; Adjunct Professor of Criminology, Marquette University; and Director, Center for Forensic Psychiatry and Risk Assessment, Milwaukee, WI

Humana Press
Totowa, New Jersey

999 Riverview Drive, Suite 208
Totowa, New Jersey 07512
humanapress.com

This publication is printed on acid-free paper. ∞

ANSI Z39.48-1984 (American Standards Institute) Permanence of Paper for Printed Library Materials.

Production editor: Robin B. Weisberg

Cover design by Patricia F. Cleary.

For additional copies, pricing for bulk purchases, and/or information about other Humana titles, contact Humana at the above address or at any of the following numbers: Tel.: 973-256-1699; Fax: 973-256-8341; E-mail: orders@humanapr.com; or visit our Website: www.humanapress.com

Printed in the United States of America. 10 9 8 7 6 5 4 3 2 1
Kocsis, Richard N.
Criminal profiling : principles and practice / Richard N. Kocsis.
p. cm.
Includes bibliographical references and index.
ISBN 1-58829-639-3 (alk. paper)
1. Criminal behavior, Prediction of. 2. Criminal investigation--Psychological aspects.
3. Violent offenders--Psychology. I. Title.
HV8073.5.K63 2006
363.2'32--dc22

2006014229

Dedication

Per là mia bella principessa, Rosanna. Szeretlek tiszta szivembol.

Foreword

After a sharp increase in the mid-1990s, crime in general, with the exception of homicide, has decreased in the past several years. Nevertheless, the investigative abilities and stamina of police officers in many agencies continue to be taxed and overwhelmed. Among crimes, the most difficult to solve have been and are those that are often repetitive or serial in nature, such as murder, rape, and arson. The consequences of these crimes are frequently appalling and create a profound uneasiness in the community. In an attempt to improve the clearance rate of existing investigative methods, criminological scholars have devised theoretical systems and specific techniques to facilitate the identification and apprehension of these serial offenders. Often these offenders are clever, astute criminals who challenge the investigative police and derive pleasure from doing so.

The systems, which have sprouted worldwide (e.g., Australia, England, Canada, the United States), are termed *profiling* and the various techniques *criminal profiling*. Criminal profiling is the process of observation and reflection based on the analysis of evidence collected at a crime scene. The technique of profiling aims at identifying and interpreting crime behavior or actions for the purpose of predicting the personality of the offender, his or her *modus operandi* and, possibly, motivations for the crime. The purpose of profiling is, however, not only to obtain a possible identification of important offender characteristics, but also to prevent the repetition of similar future crimes.

Richard N. Kocsis, the author of *Criminal Profiling: Principles and Practice*, is an eminent scholar in the field of criminological profiling. He has put together in a clear, concise, and easily understandable manner the historical development of his own research, which led to the conceptualization of his profiling method—Crime Action Profiling (CAP)—that he distinguishes from other types of profiling. He thoroughly explains his research efforts in assessing the accuracy of profiling and the pragmatic aspect of his own method. He points out the underlying psychological mechanisms operating in serial crimes and highlights the utilitarian perspective of his profiling method.

One of the difficulties for practical criminologists is the application of theory to practice and, in the case of criminal profiling, the construction of the actual profiles, which often has been relegated to a restricted group of scholars. After having explained his concept of criminal profiling and the utilitarian perspective of his method, supported by his numerous studies, Dr. Kocsis guides the reader step by step in the construction of a criminal profile, inclusive of a geographical profile. Indeed, within the umbrella of his CAP approach, he is focused on developing a set of generic principles for the construction of a profile. Thus, he shares his acquired knowledge with others. The importance of this book is found not only in its clear, unambiguous narrative, but in the didactic, vulgarized method used by Dr. Kocsis, which helps the noninitiated understand the process of profiling and the initiated to put it into practice. In so doing, he overcomes what is often seen as the obstrusity of criminal profiling.

In *Criminal Profiling: Principles and Practice*, Dr. Kocsis, shows that he has the unusual capacity to simplify the difficult. That is what a real scholar does.

George B. Palermo, *MD, MScCrim*
Clinical Professor of Psychiatry and Neurology, Medical College of Wisconsin; Adjunct Professor of Criminology, Marquette University; and Director, Center for Forensic Psychiatry and Risk Assessment, Milwaukee, WI

Preface

The Evolution of Crime Action Profiling

As a forensic psychologist, most topics involving the interaction of the criminal justice system with the science of psychology interest me. It was not until the start of the 1990s, however, that I first learned of a fascinating and purportedly new technique whereby police investigators could develop a description of an offender based not on any witness report, but on behaviors evidently displayed during the commission of a crime. What captured my attention most about this technique was the context in which it was applied. Often, work and research in the domain of forensic psychology considers issues in a reactive context. Examples include psychological evaluations of an individual for the purpose of an insanity defense or a person's potential for recidivism in the context of a parole hearing. Here, however, was something that could be used in a proactive context, while a criminal investigation was still very much afoot. The disciplinary knowledge of psychology could in this sense be used to compile a description of the likely offender to assist with an on-going investigation. This remarkable concept or investigative tool as police referred to it was simply referred to as psychological profiling. I quickly learned, however, that although the underlying concept surrounding this technique was the same, the title assigned to it varied markedly depending on differing practitioners and their disciplinary backgrounds, which was often reflected in the nomenclature adopted by these practitioners. The terms criminal profiling, offender profiling, criminal investigative analysis, and criminal personality profiling all seemed to be used interchangeably to describe the practice. With this new awareness (of what I will for the sake of simplicity refer to here as "profiling"), I set about collecting, reading, and learning as much as I could about the technique. Initially, I was thoroughly captivated by the material. The prospect of being able to deduce the identity of a criminal and thereby assist in the investigation of violent crime was of great interest to me and, I considered, of enormous practical benefit to law enforcement agencies throughout the world. However, after about 6 months of exploring the available literature doubts began to creep into my mind as I contemplated the research on the topic.

First, I started to perceive similarities between supposedly original independent studies and their respective data pools. It appeared to me that some articles did not actually report a study in a holistic manner as it had been undertaken. Instead, a study frequently appeared divided into smaller components. This subdivision seemed to enhance the number of publications and exposure gained from what appeared to me to be essentially a single study. Although subdivision *per se* is not wrong, it should, in my view be more of a rarity than a common practice and should be clearly acknowledged so that the context and origin of the data are clearly made known.

Also of significance to me was the originality of the samples gathered for the purpose of a study and the publications generated from these samples. Cognizant of the comparatively low volume of serial violent crimes that form the basis of the bulk of profiling research, I assumed the collection of samples would be difficult to obtain and therefore scarce in number. In contrast to this assumption I was surprised by the number of available studies emanating from what I expected to be a very limited data pool from any given country. There is an expression known as double-dipping that serves to describe an inelegant practice of repetition or recycling. The term arose from the distasteful practice of a person contaminating a shared food receptacle by re-dipping a piece of bread, for example, that had already been dipped and gnawed on into a fondue bowl shared by others. In a somewhat analogous capacity, I could not help but wonder about some original studies and whether the same data was simply being re-analyzed or double-dipped by different researchers who held some common affiliation with the source of the data. The net effect of these observations with respect to the published literature was the realization that the published material could easily create the impression that a substantial corpus of research existed on the topic of profiling when perhaps only a smaller amount of truly original material existed.

The second issue that came to my attention involved the content and application of some of the published literature. A large proportion seemed to focus more on describing and discussing profiling and its potential uses rather than systematically explaining how a criminal profile was or should be constructed. Granted, some original empirical studies have been undertaken that offer interesting offender typologies that appear valid and relevant to profiling. The systematic interpretation and application of this information, however, remained something of a mystery. This gap in the literature served to highlight, to my mind, the divide between the "art" dimension of profiling and the "science" of profiling. Even today, there exists debate about whether the practice of profiling is in reality an art or a science. Indeed, in one sense profiling can be viewed as both. The scientific aspect of profiling it seems is well catered for in a number of studies that have produced a range of taxonomies for different types of behaviors and offenders. This literature, however, is often silent on how such categories should be systematically interpreted and applied to any given circumstance for the purpose of formulating a profile. In the absence of such exposition the art dimension to profiling has evolved.

A third issue of concern to me was determining what was the likely accuracy of profiling in correctly predicting the characteristics of an unknown offender. Despite this being a seemingly fundamental issue, I was surprised by the scarcity of what I would regard as robust evidence. At the time, the predominant source of material describing the accuracy of profiles and their utility were anecdotal accounts from profilers themselves. While the analogous use of clinical vignettes are common in the consideration of mental disorders and their treatment within the disciplines of psychiatry and psychology such vignettes exist alongside an equal if not greater number of carefully crafted studies within such disciplines that empirically and impartially seek to evaluate the effectiveness of such treatments. Despite the ever-growing popularity and apparent optimism surrounding the use of profiling that appears to characterize much of the literature, equivalent scientifically grounded trials of profiling were to my mind, remarkably conspicuous by their absence.

The defining moment for me, however, perhaps arrived when I was consulted about a high-profile serial murder case. The police investigators had, in respect of another serial murder case, consulted expert profilers from an internationally renowned law enforcement agency only a few years earlier. The procured profile did not seem to logically accord with Australia's population demographics. Consequently, on this investigation different tactics were employed and police consulted numerous sources (including myself) to see what assistance could be provided. With an artificial sense of confidence derived from my knowledge of the literature, I set about carefully examining and considering the circumstances of the case and the questions that were posed to me. From the outset, I found that the details surrounding the murders seldom comfortably or neatly matched the evident categories and patterns described in the published literature. For example, although one tantalizing similarity was clearly apparent between the case under consideration and the research literature, the matching features were derived from the research developed in the context of rapists, not serial murderers. Although behaviors at times were evident that matched one distinct offender category, matching behaviors inherent to another dichotomously opposite category were also similarly evident. Before long, I found myself mixing the research literature with my own clinical knowledge wherever I perceived some relevance. I was duly thanked for my efforts, but despite this I couldn't help but wonder how useful my ideas had truly been or whether they genuinely offered anything more than what could have been deduced through common sense. It was these doubts about the research literature at the time, combined with my own experience in constructing a profile, that led me to contemplate the full extent of the deficit that existed between the reputation and the capabilities of profiling. It was from this time I realized that far more work and research was required into criminal profiling.

Today, with the luxury of hindsight, the development of profiling can be seen as akin to the field of personality theory. Within the disciplines of psychology and psychiatry, there exists an accepted consensus in the existence of a conceptual construct known as the mind. Although there is common agreement in the concept of the mind, there are numerous rival approaches or theories that attempt to explain the nature and operation of the mind. A few examples of these differing approaches or "personality theories" include the psychoanalytic, behaviorist, and biological theories. The work and research into profiling can be viewed in an analogous fashion. There appears to be a general consensus that profiling is a concept whereby crime behaviors can be interpreted for the purpose of making predictions concerning the probable offender's characteristics. Akin to the varying personality theories, differing approaches have evolved over time that propose how crime behaviors are interpreted or profiled. In drawing this analogy with respect to the development of profiling, it is important to appreciate what roughly constitutes or equates with an approach to the profiling of certain crimes. In this context an approach can be loosely conceived as a coherent body of work or research composed of a number of original studies that commonly share some distinctive theoretical or methodological basis concerning the profiling of a variety of crimes.*

Arguably, the first and oldest approach to profiling emerged when individual mental health professionals were consulted to assist in criminal investigations involving often bizarre and seemingly unsolvable crimes. Historical examples of such consultations span back many decades and include now infamous consultations such as Dr. Thomas Bond in 1888 in the investigation of the Whitechappel murders (also known as Jack the Ripper) and Dr. James

*It should be noted that although not meeting my adopted definition of an approach, scholars including Bruce Arrigo, Steven Egger, Eric Hickey, Jack Levin, and Louis Schlesinger (to name only a few) have each made valuable contributions to the topic of profiling and/or serial violent crime.

Brussel in the 1940–1950s investigation of the Mad Bomber of New York. Although admittedly lacking an original body of research on the specific topic of profiling, there is nonetheless some clear commonality among these individuals, which is perhaps founded in the disciplinary knowledge and training they share. Namely, their efforts in relating their knowledge of psychiatry/psychology/criminology and clinical experience to the profiling of a crime. This example of profiling has come to be known as Diagnostic Evaluation (DE) and in many respects it arguably still represents the most common and readily accessible approach to profiling violent crimes *(1)*. These historical antecedents serve to dispel myths concerning the comparatively recent invention of profiling by any individual or law enforcement organization. They indicate that the concept of criminal profiling in predicting the probable characteristics of a perpetrator of a violent crime is neither new nor revolutionary.

Such DEs served to inspire the development of another approach to profiling now commonly referred to as Criminal Investigative Analysis (CIA). This approach comprises the collective works of the FBI's Behavioral Science Unit *(2)*. Although the research underpinning CIA does not support the invention of profiling by the FBI, it does nonetheless represent the first cogent body of research to specifically and systematically consider the profiling of violent crimes. Additionally, the efforts of the FBI through CIA can be credited for popularizing the concept of profiling among law enforcement agencies throughout the world. This popularization in itself is a significant accomplishment that should not be underestimated or devalued as without these efforts it is debatable to what extent, if at all, the practice of profiling would have evolved beyond the classical circumstance of DE.

Perceived inadequacies with the various approaches to profiling provided the impetus for the development of other approaches. In this respect, the underlying ideology behind CIA was no exception. Although inspired by the DE efforts of clinicians such as Dr. Brussel *(2)*, researchers in the FBI Behavioral Science Unit were dissatisfied with the clinical/treatment perspectives of DE. Accordingly, CIA set about developing a method of profiling that specifically catered to the needs of law enforcement personnel in the investigation of violent crime. In particular, CIA attempted to develop a pragmatic method for the profiling of crimes that would be readily accessible and comprehensible to police personnel. The pursuit of this objective led to research that considered the profiling of violent crimes as a technique informed by various investigative concepts or maxims. These maxims were derived from various offender typologies developed by the FBI's Behavioral Science Unit through their own original studies of incarcerated offenders. Possibly the most renowned of these typologies being the organized–disorganized dichotomy with its underlying maxim of the interpretation of crimes by the level of behavioral sophistication exhibited at a crime scene.

Perceived dissatisfaction with the typologies and concomitant investigative maxims inherent to CIA in part led to the development of another approach—Investigative Psychology (IP). IP sought to approach the concept of profiling from a stronger methodological basis indicative of research practices common to the social sciences. Once again, a number of original studies were undertaken of various offender groups typically via the use of archival data sources such as closed police cases. Results from these studies were interpreted more in terms of ideographic themes that were argued to be indicative of the offenders who committed the examined crimes. Thus, the commission of a murder, for example, was argued to be interpretable dependent on the presence or absence of semi-dichotomous themes of whether there was an instrumental or expressive purpose inherent to the commission of the crime. Possibly the most distinctive ideological feature of the research conducted under the banner of IP was its conceptualization of profiling as a psychological subdiscipline seemingly distinct from mainstream forensic psychology. This disciplinary splinter appears manifest in the nomenclature adopted to describe the research undertaken and the availability of tertiary qualifications in the field of IP.

Another recent body of thought which can be viewed as an approach to profiling is that of Behavior Evidence Analysis (BEA). There are, however, some significant limitations in describing BEA as a distinct approach to profiling as it does not appear to be informed by a discrete substantive body of original empirical research. Instead, what BEA offers in some respects is a fusion of previous criminological literature on various forms of violent crime, the forensic sciences and philosophical concepts related to modes of reasoning, most notably, inductive vs deductive reasoning. BEA seems to hypothesize that a method of analysis is possible, whereby crimes may be interpreted for the purpose of profiling by adopting deductive reasoning processes as opposed to inductive ones. Given our current understanding of how the human mind functions and cognitively processes information in a heterogeneous fashion, some inherent difficulties exist with such a hypothesis *(3)*.

Nonetheless, BEA is noteworthy for one reason in particular. The invention of BEA arose from perceived dissatisfaction, albeit perhaps mistakenly at times, with other profiling approaches which seemed preoccupied with the statistical generation of aggregated profiles. BEA identifies and warns of the very real dangers of criminal profiles that adopt a colloquial "one-size-fits-all" approach in relying on conceptualizations of the typical offender instead of adequately considering the circumstances of each crime and the potential uniqueness of its perpetrator. Thus, BEA highlights the need for profiling methods to be, wherever possible, flexible in their capacity to account for various combinations of individual factors concerning a particular crime and advocates the generation of criminal profiles specifically based on such unique factors.

It is against this backdrop that I have written this book more than a decade and a half later. Much has transpired since I first learned of profiling and immersed myself in the literature on the topic. Indeed, I have conducted many of my own studies in the area. Akin to all of the other approaches to profiling the impetus for my own research efforts has been my dissatisfaction with the available literature and the methods advocated. The volume, scope, and methodology employed in the studies that I have undertaken over the years have developed to such an extent that I view them as forming a distinct approach to profiling in itself which I refer to as Crime Action Profiling (CAP).

CAP adopts the view that profiling essentially represents a psychological technique that has its foundations in the disciplinary knowledge of forensic psychology. As can be seen by the historical development of profiling from its DE origins, profiling was a task within the repertoire of functions traditionally performed by psychiatrists or psychologists who were consulted by police investigators to assist in bizarre and seemingly unsolvable crimes. Over time, the growth in the popularity of profiling led to its practice by a range of other professionals such as police officers, criminologists and social scientists. In this respect the ideology inherent to CAP deviates from that of both CIA and IP. That is, CAP adopts the view that profiling is simply a technique that originates from the discipline of forensic psychology.* As a consequence, this conception of profiling assumes knowledge of human behavior and psychology such as personality dynamics and human psychopathologies.# This differs from CIA, which posits profiling as an investigative technique more within the corpus of knowledge and domain of law enforcement, and IP, which postures

*In defining this conceptualization of profiling, it should be noted that although CAP views profiling as a technique within the disciplinary boundaries of forensic psychology, this conception relates to the corpus of scientific knowledge associated with forensic psychology. It is not meant to imply that the construction of profiles should be restricted to forensic psychologists *per se*, but rather, the body of scientific knowledge that comprises profiling should be viewed as traditionally within the topic domain of forensic psychology.

#In this regard, knowledge of human behavior and psychology is conceived as a distinct body of knowledge which, it is argued, is a closely related prerequisite to profiling. Akin to disciplinary knowledge of the forensic sciences the reader is assumed to possess this knowledge for the purpose of this book.

that profiling has evolved to such an extent that its conceptualization is worthy of forming a discrete psychological discipline unto itself.

How CAP conceives and characterizes profiling as a technique within the existing disciplinary boundaries of forensic psychology is important for another reason. In addition to the study of mental disease, the discipline of psychology also expends considerable effort on the study and development of practical skills related to the clinical practice or application of psychology. Examples of these include clinical interviewing techniques, assessment of clients and conventions for writing various forms of diagnostic reports. In an analogous manner the research strands of CAP have studied both the behavioral patterns inherent to violent crimes (akin to psychology's study of mental disease) as well as the structure, processes, accuracy and skills related to constructing profiles (akin to the clinical practice of psychology). This is a distinguishing feature of CAP as other approaches to profiling have predominantly focused solely on the study of offender typologies and have, for the most part, largely ignored such issues related to the practical concept of constructing a profile.

It is this ideological conception of profiling as a technique within the disciplinary domain of forensic psychology that also accounts for its nomenclature "Crime Action Profiling." The term CAP is used to help differentiate it from other tasks psychologists regularly perform. The discipline of psychology operates by applying a body of information concerning mental disorders to clients who present for a variety of reasons, the most frequent of which is psychological assessment. Within this context a discrete area of psychology known as psychometrics exists which often makes use of tools such as personality and psychological profiles. In the context of this book however, the term profiling does not refer to the evaluation of a patient, but instead the interpretation of an offender's actions that are evidenced in a crime scene and from which predictions about that offender's characteristics can be made. In this respect, the term Crime Action Profiling is used to describe and signify this process relating to the consideration of crime actions and the prediction, or profiling, of offender characteristics from those actions.

The studies canvassed throughout this book represent my own original, empirically based work on the topic of criminal profiling. Over the past decade and a half this work has been published in a range of scholarly peer-reviewed journals. Their publication in this format, however, has only served to provide a disjointed method of communicating their aggregated meaning to primarily only those who read academic journals. Consequently, in the pages of this book I have, for the first time, attempted to draw together in a systematic fashion the research I have undertaken to provide a comprehensive compendium of the research endeavors that characterize the CAP approach to the profiling of violent crimes.

Additionally, in recognition of the application of profiling in criminal investigations and the need for this material to be comprehensible to a wider audience, I have attempted to explain the many concepts in a manner that does not require the reader to possess advanced qualifications in subjects such as statistics, psychiatry, or psychology. In this regard, I have endeavored to write this book in a manner that renders it, in some respects, accessible to the intelligent lay person as well as personnel engaged in the legal, law enforcement, and criminal justice fields.

In an effort to maximize the accessibility of the CAP research contained in this book I have adopted a deliberate structure. The initial four chapters are intended to explain the implications of the body of work I have undertaken which examines the skills, accuracy, components and processes surrounding the construction of a criminal profile. As previously mentioned systematic consideration of such issues have, in my view, been gravely neglected. In Chapter 5, the focus shifts to the CAP research and methods developed for the profiling of violent crimes. The objective of Chapter 5 is to define and identify the forms of violent crime that, in my view, are most applicable to profiling. Chapter 5 also examines the types of crimes for which CAP models have been generated and which are the subject of subsequent chapters.

Chapter 6 is perhaps the most pivotal in that I have for the first time attempted to articulate a generic procedure by which the various CAP models canvassed later in Chapters 7–9 may be utilized for the practical development of a criminal profile. The primary focus of Chapter 6 is to describe a systematic method for the interpretation and use of the CAP models. Thus, Chapter 6 aims to instruct the lay person, and in particular readers who lack an appreciation of advanced statistics and/or social science methodologies on how to use the various CAP models to profile a particular crime without necessarily needing to comprehend how each model was originally built.

The subsequent three chapters (i.e., Chapters 7–9) then canvass the respective CAP studies undertaken into crimes of serial rape, serial/sexual murder and serial arson and explain how each of the models were developed. It is crucial to appreciate that the statistical and methodological expositions contained in each of these chapters are provided for readers who are primarily interested in understanding the theoretical and methodological principles incumbent to the development of each of the CAP models. In this respect, a detailed understanding of this material is not essential for readers who wish to use the models for the purpose of aiding them in the construction of a criminal profile.

The final two chapters of the book return to the objective of providing the reader with a greater understanding of the CAP research and its pragmatic application. Specifically, Chapter 10 outlines procedures for the analysis of offense spatial locations, while Chapter 11 discusses procedurally how to develop a written criminal profile.

The work of CAP that is discussed throughout this book is cognizant of the purpose of profiling in assisting criminal investigations and is therefore predominantly focused on crimes that, in my view, will most directly and frequently benefit from the input of a criminal profile. CAP firmly advocates the scientific development of profiling and incorporates social science principles into its methods. The CAP principles recognize the dangers in being heavily reliant on standardized templates of offenders and instead advocates for malleable mechanisms in accounting for the individual circumstances of a given crime wherever possible.

I have embarked on many objectives in writing this book, but if the reader considers my combined efforts to have increased his or her understanding of criminal profiling and how it works, I will be content.

Richard N. Kocsis, PhD

References

1. Wilson, P.R., Lincoln, R., & Kocsis, R.N. (1997). Validity, utility and ethics of profiling for serial violent and sexual offenders. Psychiatry, Psychology and Law, 4, 1–12.
2. Innes, B. (2003). Profile of a criminal mind. Leicester: Silverdale Books.
3. Kocsis, R.N. & Palermo, G.B. (2005). Ten major problems with criminal profiling. American Journal of Forensic Psychiatry, 26(2), 45–67.

Contents

About the Author

Richard N. Kocsis, BA (Hons) *Psych*, Cert Man, MCrim, PhD *Psych* is a forensic psychologist in private practice. He is the author of more than 80 scholarly articles, and 2 books on the topics of criminal profiling, serial violent offenders and their criminal investigation, and is currently producing an edited book series also in this area. He has served as an expert consultant to law enforcement, emergency and prosecution agencies, as well as private law firms. In addition to his clinical and forensic work, he has held various academic positions in the areas of forensic psychology and criminology, including Lecturer in Investigations (Policing). In 2000, he was awarded the Australian Museum's prestigious *Eureka* prize for critical thinking in recognition of his scientific research in the area of criminal profiling.

Chapter 1

What Is Criminal Profiling?

Summary

Within the context of this book, the concept of *criminal profiling* is defined and described as a technique whereby the probable characteristics of a criminal offender or offenders are predicted based on the behaviors exhibited in the commission of a crime. A brief overview of the historical antecedents and development of criminal profiling is also presented and illustrates that criminal profiling is conceptually old and indicative of the human race's long-held fascination with the assessment and prediction of criminality. This chapter concludes by outlining some of the common applications and objectives of criminal profiles.

Key Words: Criminal profiling; definitions; history; objectives; applications.

Introduction

Unfortunately, the term *criminal profiling* has, at times, come to be understood as meaning different things, and part of the confusion arises from the different nomenclature used often interchangeably, including offender profiling, criminal personality profiling, investigative profiling, and psychological profiling. Descriptions of criminal profiling have included "a collection of leads" *(1)* and a "biological sketch of behavioral patterns, trends, and tendencies" *(2)*. More detailed descriptions of criminal profiling, however, include the following:

> *A forensic technique which seeks to provide investigative agencies with specific information which will help focus attention on individuals with personality traits that parallel traits of other perpetrators who have committed similar other offenses. (3, p. 236)*

or

The process of identifying personality traits, behavioral tendencies, and demographic variables of an offender based on characteristics of the crime. (4, p. 167)

More recent descriptions of profiling have suggested the following:

Criminal profiling refers to the process of identifying personality traits, behavioral tendencies, geographic locations and demographic or biological descriptors of an offender based on characteristics of the crime. (5, p. 186)

...an attempt to provide investigators with more information on a serial murderer who is yet to be identified. (6, p. 193)

Irrespective of the particular descriptions used, at their most basic level, all effectively attempt to describe the same underlying concept. That is, criminal profiling represents a process whereby behaviors and/or actions exhibited in a crime are assessed and interpreted to form predictions concerning the characteristics of the probable perpetrator(s) of the crime. The composite predicted characteristics are often referred to as a criminal profile, the purpose of which is to assist investigators, typically police personnel, in the identification and thus apprehension of an unknown criminal or criminals. For simplicity, and in an attempt to minimize further confusion throughout the remainder of this book, the term *criminal profiling* or simply *profiling* is adopted here.

Having provided some exposition of what criminal profiling is, it is also important to identify and distinguish such profiling from other similarly described concepts. Criminal profiling and criminal profiles within the context of this book should not be confused with aggregated profiles that are also sometimes referred to as racial profiles or racial profiling. Criminal profiling in the context of this book refers to the systematic analysis of an individual crime or related series of crimes for the purpose of constructing a profile that describes the various characteristics of the offender likely to have committed the crime(s) specifically under examination. The use of criminal profiling commonly arises in the context of an on-going criminal investigation into a crime or crime series. Racial profiles, on the other hand, represent aggregated demographic templates of the typical type of individual who is believed to commit certain forms of crime *(7)*. One way of appreciating the distinction between racial and criminal profiles arises from the context in which they are used. For example, racial profiles may be relied on by customs services or casinos as guides for identifying, respectively, a likely drug trafficker or card-counting gambler. Based on this information, customs officers or casino investigators may select and search travelers or focus surveillance on certain players or casino patrons.

Similarly, the term *criminal profile* within the context of this book should not be confused with intelligence-based profiles of individuals that are often compiled by police and other law enforcement and intelligence organizations *(8)*. Although "intelligence" profiles contain demographic information pertaining to a particular individual, it should be recognized that these profiles frequently represent a compilation of known and suspected particulars regarding a specific individual who may have been previously apprehended, wanted, or strongly suspected of having committed an offense or offenses. It should also be noted that criminal profiles within the context of this book are also distinct from DNA profiles that represent the DNA coding for some item of organic matter. The use of DNA profiles relates to the discipline of forensic science and involves the matching of DNA samples taken from a suspect with those found at the scene of a crime to establish whether they are likely to originate from the offender *(9)*.

Finally, criminal profiles are distinct from personality or psychological profiles *(10)*. Although criminal profiling is sourced in the disciplinary knowledge of psychology and is still frequently referred to as psychological profiling in some quarters, it must be understood that psychological or personality profiles within the clinical practice of psychology often refers to the evaluation and diagnosis of a presenting patient *(11)*. In contrast, criminal profiling does not relate to the examination of a presenting patient. Rather, it is the examination of a crime to interpret the behaviors evident in the commission of that crime and from an analysis of those behaviors generate a description of the individual likely to have exhibited those behaviors.

The Origins of Criminal Profiling

Contrary to media portrayals of criminal profiling as a recent or revolutionary concept, the notion of predicting the characteristics of a criminal based on the criminal's exhibited behaviors, is symbolic of the human race's long-held fascination with classifying and predicting criminality. One of the earliest examples comes from the classic poet Homer who described the character of Thersities in *The Illiad* as an ugly and malformed man whose personality was most likely indicative of a criminal disposition. The ancient philosopher Plato also suggested in his writings *Hippias Major* that ugliness was a sign of ontological imperfections and a deficit of rationality *(12)*. Similar notions of a relationship existing between anatomy and criminality have persisted throughout history and essentially culminated in the emergence of phrenology and most prominently, the writings of the Italian criminologist Cesare Lombroso *(13)*. Although these anatomically based conceptions have long since been discarded *(14,15)* the underlying conception that behavior is in some capacity a reflection of personality has remained and indeed forms one of the cornerstones of the modern-day science of psychology *(16)*.

Interestingly, one of the earliest applications of the symbiosis between behavior and personality in the context of a criminal investigation emerges from the time of Victorian England. It is often opined that truth is stranger than fiction and it seems the history of criminal profiling is demonstrative of this. Although early fictional examples of profiling date back to the novels of Sir Arthur Conan Doyle and the infamous character Sherlock Holmes *(17)*, one notable factual example of profiling relates to one of history's earliest and possibly most notorious serial killers. Presented with a series of seemingly random, sadistic, and unsolvable murders of women in the Whitechapel region, London's Criminal Investigation Division in 1888 sought the assistance of the physician Dr. Thomas Bond *(18)*. This series of murders would later become legendary and the perpetrator known as Jack the Ripper. Akin to contemporary circumstances surrounding the practice of criminal profiling, Dr. Bond was consulted to examine the available evidence concerning the case. It was thought that Dr. Bond, drawing on his professional skills and clinical expertise, could proffer some suggestions concerning the individual(s) likely to have committed the murders. Notable components of Dr. Bond's report included evaluations of the behaviors exhibited during the commission of the murders. For instance:

> *...all five murders were no doubt committed by the same hand. In the first four the throats appear to have been cut from left to right, in the last case owing to the extensive mutilation it is impossible to say in what direction the fatal cut was made. All the circumstances surrounding the murders lead me to form the opinion that the women must have been lying down when murdered. (19, p. 114)*

Also included were predictions concerning the perpetrator's probable characteristics:

> *...In each case the mutilation was implicated by a person who had no scientific nor anatomical knowledge. In my opinion he does not even possess the technical knowledge of a butcher or horse slaughterer or any person accustomed to cutting up dead animals. (19, p. 115)*

> *...A man subject to periodical attacks of Homicidal and Erotic mania. The murderer in external appearance is quite likely to be a quiet inoffensive looking man, probably middle-aged and neatly and respectably dressed. He would be solitary and eccentric in his habits, also he is most likely to be a man without regular occupation, but with a small income or pension. (19, p. 115)*

What is perhaps most startling about Dr. Bond's evaluations of the murders is that despite his comments having been originally written approximately

120 years ago, the items of information canvassed in the report closely parallel those found in many criminal profiles today. Dr. Bond's report, or the criminal profile of Jack the Ripper, attempts to evaluate the relationship between each of the murders and whether they were indeed perpetrated by the same individual. This is then followed by some discussion and analysis of the *modus operandi* adopted in killing the victims. In his report, Dr. Bond also articulates a series of features that he believes describe the characteristics of the offender, including the perpetrator's likely age, gender, manner of dress, demeanor, vocational history, and psychopathologies. Although the case of the Whitechapel murderer remains unsolved and thus prevents any meaningful evaluation of the value of Dr. Bond's profile, this early historical example highlights that the fundamental concept of criminal profiling and the core tenets of what typically comprises a criminal profile are, in truth, remarkably old.

Another notable historical example of profiling emerged in 1943 with the consultation of Dr. Walter Langer by the US Office of Strategic Services (the precursor to the contemporary CIA) for the purpose of a psychological evaluation of Adolf Hitler *(20)*. Although this profile was not undertaken within the traditional context of a criminal investigation (there can be little doubt that Hitler was indeed a notorious criminal), the assessment nonetheless sought to evaluate and predict behavioral patterns similar to those found in criminal profiles today. Specific among the questions posed to Dr. Langer was Hitler's likely reaction if confronted with the possibility of defeat. Although Dr. Langer nominated a number of potential reactions, he nonetheless astutely identified that Hitler's most likely reaction would be to commit suicide rather than face the humiliation of possible capture and trial for his actions. In light of Hitler's ultimate fate, Dr. Langer's prediction proved insightful.

Despite such historical examples, what can arguably be viewed as the progenitor of contemporary criminal profiling emerged in the 1950s with the work of Dr. James Brussel, a psychiatrist whose apparent skills in evaluating crimes led to his being consulted on a number of infamous cases *(21)*. Chief among these was Brussel's involvement in a series of bombings that plagued the city of New York and were dubbed the work of the Mad Bomber of New York. In circumstances reminiscent of the use of criminal profiles today, police investigators consulted Dr. Brussel to construct a criminal profile of the offender who had eluded apprehension and whose bombing campaign had been underway for many years. After considering the available case materials on the bombings, Dr. Brussel constructed a profile that identified numerous characteristics that were subsequently found to match the attributes of the bomber George Metesky when eventually apprehended *(21)*. However, Dr.

Brussel's efforts were distinguished by the remarkable perspicuity he demonstrated in identifying some of Metesky's characteristics. Most notable among the predicted features was Brussel's conclusion that the bomber would be a fastidiously neat individual. This, he reasoned, was manifest in a number of behavioral attributes surrounding the crimes, such as the apparent care the bomber demonstrated in drafting letters to the authorities when seeking to communicate and explain his actions. In this respect, Dr. Brussel indicated that the bomber was likely to be a neatly presented individual who would most likely prefer blue double-breasted suits that would probably be worn with the jacket buttons fastened. The bomber, Metesky, was apprehended late one evening at his home. Before leaving, Metesky was permitted to change out of his pajamas before being formally taken into custody. In line with Brussel's predictions, Metesky was neatly presented and changed into a blue double-breasted suit, which he wore with all the buttons fastened *(21)*.

It was in part the remarkable insights of Dr. Brussel in the case of the Mad Bomber of New York and the Boston Strangler case *(22)* that inspired the research and development of criminal profiling by the FBI's Behavioral Science Unit *(23)*. At approximately the same time, numerous other individual scholars concerned with the phenomenon of serial violent crime also investigated the concept of profiling *(5,6,24–26)*. With the seemingly growing prevalence of serial violent crime, interest in the concept of profiling gained momentum and led to the development of other formalized schools of thought on the topic.

The Structure, Applications, and Objectives of Criminal Profiles

Describing the precise objectives and structure of criminal profiles is not straightforward, partly because of the differing disciplinary perspectives surrounding the technique and partly because of the ever-developing and diversifying conceptions of the practice. Despite variations, some underlying consensus can nonetheless be discerned. For the most part, a criminal profile consists of information that predominantly serves to describe the biographical features of the probable perpetrator(s) of a crime. Thus, criminal profiles typically contain information about the probable offender concerning the following:

- Likely demographics, such as age and gender.
- Legal history, including any antecedence (i.e., history of prior criminal offenses/convictions).
- Vocational background (i.e., the work the offender is likely to be engaged in, if any).

- Family characteristics (i.e., the likely background of the offender's family).
- Habits and social interests (sports, hobbies, or other interests that the offender may have).
- Mode of transport (type of vehicle, if any, the offender has).
- Various personality characteristics (the offender's demeanor, appearance, etc).

In addition to such biographical information, it should be noted that criminal profiles frequently also include information pertaining to the approximate location of an offender's residence. This type of information is often the product of what is now commonly referred to as *geographic profiling (27,28).* Although some arguments exist for the formulation of a discrete discipline known as geographic profiling, the basis for these arguments appear to be largely sourced in vocational interests. Although some research developments have indeed emerged in the evaluation of geographic features relevant to criminal profiling, information such as an offender's likely area of residence have long been components of the information typically contained in criminal profiles *(1,29).* Consequently, although a separate set of methods exist for the evaluation of such geographic information (*see* Chapter 10), it is preferable to view these methods as simply a subcomponent of information that comprises a criminal profile.

In describing the application of criminal profiles, it must be emphasized that contrary to many fictional media portrayals, criminal profiles by themselves do not solve crimes *(30,31).* Instead, criminal profiling is best viewed as a resource that can be used to assist a criminal investigation when conventional methods employed have stalled or even failed to identify the perpetrator *(32–34).* This circumstance frequently arises when the offender possesses some form of aberrant drive and/or psychopathology *(3)* and thus the motives, traditionally used by investigators to make deductions about a given perpetrator, are not clearly evident *(35,36).*

To date, the research literature indicates that criminal profiles have been found to be most effective as an adjunct to traditional investigative techniques and not as a stand-alone solution for the resolution of specific crimes *(37,38).* Thus, criminal profiles represent a device by which an investigation may focus its resources and lines of inquiry. In this respect, criminal profiles do not, under any circumstance, serve as a substitute for conventional procedures typically undertaken in criminal investigations.

As previously mentioned, defining the objectives of a criminal profile is once again largely dependent on the adopted ideological perspective. Indeed, many of these variations appear to be grounded in attempts to expand the disciplinary boundaries of what constitutes criminal profiling and occasionally, it seems, the services that may be rendered by an individual who operates under the title of profiler. Indeed, it is worthy to note that many of these variations appear highly derivative of work and research undertaken in other topic areas or separate disciplines altogether. Some examples include interrogation and/or interview suggestions in police questioning and judicial proceedings *(39)*, crisis negotiation tactics *(31)*, equivocal death assessments *(40)*, and even decision-making models on how investigative lines of inquiry should be followed. Irrespective of these variations, there nonetheless appears to be some general consensus concerning the two core themes that appear to be associated with the technique of criminal profiling:

- To provide a descriptive template of the features that characterize the probable perpetrator(s) of a particular crime(s) under investigation.
- To provide tactical suggestions on how facets of a criminal investigation may be undertaken.

Although the first objective is self-explanatory and in many respects characterizes the information inherent to a criminal profile, the second objective is more of an elaboration on how information contained in a profile could potentially be used during the course of an investigation. The range of possible tactics concerning how information contained in a profile may be used is very much dependent on the particular circumstances of the crime under investigation as well as the ingenuity and innovation of the consultant profiler. On this score it should be noted that many of the controversies related to criminal profiling have involved highly unethical, unprofessional, and sometimes even unlawful tactical applications of criminal profiles *(33,41,42)*. Some of the more conventional applications of criminal profiles are listed here:

- A guide for how to potentially identify suspect(s) to the crime under investigation.
- A guide for how to prioritize/focus investigative lines of inquiry on existing suspects.
- A guide for patrol policing operations to potentially reduce the commission of further offenses.
- A guide for possible surveillance operations.
- A guide for search and seizure operations.

Finally, it should be clearly understood that criminal profiles are incapable of identifying the exact perpetrator of a crime. Although material in Chapter 4 will examine the specific forms of information that profilers appear most adept in identifying, it is unlikely that the accuracy of criminal profiling will evolve to such an extent that an offender's exact identity can be predicted. Instead, the information inherent to profiles will most probably remain within the realm of probabilities in describing features that are likely to characterize the individual most likely responsible for the offense(s). Consequently, it must always be understood that despite concerted efforts, criminal profiling will always involve a margin of speculation and error.

Conclusion

It should be apparent from this chapter that defining *criminal profiling* is not as straightforward as one might expect. Part of the difficulty lies in the apparent popularity of the term *profiling* and the different connotations it seems to have acquired within criminal justice/investigative realms. Another problem stems from the differing perspectives and tasks rivaling schools of thought conceive as inherent to the technique of criminal profiling. Despite these differences, some consensus can be discerned in the sense that criminal profiling is a process whereby exhibited criminal behaviors are evaluated for the purpose of making some prediction concerning the characteristics of the probable offender. The common purpose of a criminal profile is to provide information to assist in the criminal investigation of seemingly intractable serial/sexual violent crimes. Although the concept of criminal profiling has been popularized as a somewhat revolutionary concept, the underlying premise is, in truth, remarkably old and indicative of a fascination humans have always held in trying to understand and predict criminality.

References

1. Rossi, D. (1982). Crime scene behavioral analysis: Another tool for the law enforcement investigator. Police Chief, 18(4),152–155.
2. Vorpagel, R.E. (1982). Painting psychological profiles: Charlatanism, coincidence, charisma or new science. Police Chief, 3(8), 156–159.
3. Geberth, V.J. (1983). Practical homicide investigation: Tactics, procedures and forensic techniques. Boca Raton, FL: CRC Press.
4. Bartol, C.R. and Bartol, A.M. (1994). Psychology and law. Pacific Grove, CA: Brooks/Cole.
5. Hickey, E. (2003). The encyclopaedia of murder and violent crime. Thousand Oaks, CA: Sage.
6. Egger, S. (2003). The need to kill: Inside the world of the serial killer. Upper Saddle River, NJ: Prentice-Hall.
7. Tyler, T.R. and Wakslak, C.J. (2004). Profiling and police legitimacy: Procedural justice attributions of motive, and acceptance of police authority. Criminology, 42(2), 253–281.
8. Bullock J.A., Haddow, G.D., Coppola, D., Ergin, E., Westerman, L., and Yeletaysi, S. (2005). Introduction to homeland security. London, UK: Elsevier.
9. Lazer, D., ed. (2004). DNA and the criminal justice system: The technology of justice. Boston: MIT Press.
10. Anastasi, A. (1976). Psychological testing, 4th ed. New York: Macmillan.

11. Morrison, J. (1995). DSM-IV made easy: The clinician's guide to diagnosis. New York: Guilford.
12. Woodruff, P. (1982). Hippias major/Plato. Indianapolis: Hackett.
13. Gibson, M. (2002). Born to crime: Cesare Lombroso and the origins of biological criminology. Westport, CT: Praeger.
14. Brown, S.E., Esbensen, F., and Geis, G. (1996). Criminology: Explaining crime and its context, 2nd ed. Cincinnati, OH: Anderson.
15. Jones, S. (2001). Criminology. London, UK: Butterworths.
16. Eysenck, H. and Eysenck, S.B.G. (1969). Personality structure and measurement. London: Routledge & Kegan Paul.
17. Doyle, A.C. (1891). The original illustrated Sherlock Holmes. Secaucus, NJ: Castle.
18. Rumbelow, D. (1988). The complete Jack the Ripper. London: Penguin.
19. Whittington-Egan, R. (1975). A casebook on Jack the Ripper. London: Wiley.
20. Langer, W. (1972). The mind of Adolf Hitler. New York: New American Library.
21. Brussel, J. (1968). Casebook of a criminal psychiatrist. New York: Bernard Geis.
22. Frank, G. (1966). The Boston strangler. New York: New American Library.
23. Innes, B. (2003). Profile of a criminal mind. Leicester: Silverdale Books.
24. Fox, J.A. and Levin, J. (1994). Overkill: Mass murder and serial killing exposed. New York: Plenum.
25. Hickey, E.W. (1997). Serial murderers and their victims, 2nd ed. Fresno, CA: Wadsworth.
26. Holmes, R.M. and Holmes, S.T. (1996). Profiling violent crimes: An investigative tool, 2nd ed. Thousand Oaks, CA: Sage.
27. Canter, D. (1994). Criminal shadows. London: HarperCollins.
28. Rossmo, D.K. (1997). Geographic profiling. In: Jackson, J.L. and Bekerian, D., eds. Offender profiling: Theory, research and practice. London: Wiley, pp.159–176.
29. Kind, S.S. (1987). Navigational ideas and the Yorkshire Ripper investigation. Journal of Navigation, 40, 385–393.
30. Nowikowski, F. (1995). Psychological offender profiling: An overview. The Criminologist, 19, 255–273.
31. Ressler, R.K. and Shachtman, T. (1992). Whoever fights monsters. London: Simon & Schuster.
32. Flemming, L. (1994). Serial murder. Australian Police Journal, 48(6), 59–72.
33. Jeffers, H.P. (1992). Profiles in evil. London: Warner Bros.
34. Vandiver, J. (1982). Crime profiling shows promise. Law and Order, 30(10), 33–78.
35. Fisher, A.J. (1993). Techniques of crime scene investigation, 5th ed. New York: Elsevier.
36. Walter, R. (1987). Sex killers: Their actions and reactions. Australian Police Journal, 34(2), 92–97.
37. Jackson, J.L, Van Hoppen, P.J., and Hebrink, J. (1993). Does the service meet the needs? Amsterdam: Netherlands Institute for the Study of Criminality.
38. Pinizzotto, A.J. (1984). Forensic psychology: Criminal personality profiling. Journal of Police Science and Administration, 12(1), 32–40.
39. Douglas, J.E. and Olshaker, M. (1995). Mindhunter. New York: Scribner.

40. Hazelwood, R.R., Dietz, P.E., and Burgess, A.W. (1982). Sexual fatalities: Behavioral reconstruction in equivocal cases. Journal of Forensic Science, 127, 763–773.
41. Kocsis, R.N. and Coleman, S. (2000). The unexplored ethics of criminal psychological profiling. In: Godwin, M., ed. Criminal psychology and forensic technology: A collaborative approach to effective profiling. New York: CRC Press, pp. 202–219.
42. Crace, J. (1995). Inside the criminal mind. New Statesman and Society, 29–30.

Chapter 2

Smoke and Mirrors

*The Illusions of Accuracy in Criminal Profiles**

Summary

The technique of criminal profiling has proliferated over recent decades, despite a remarkable lack of empirically rigorous evidence concerning its accuracy. Notwithstanding the absence of evidence, the very circumstance of the continued use of profiles by police investigators is often regarded as proof of their accuracy. This phenomenon is essentially informed by an "operational utilitarian argument." Namely, anecdotal evaluations of criminal profiles sponsor their continued use. This chapter is concerned with a series of empirical studies that systematically test the reliability of such anecdotal evaluations concerning the perceived accuracy of criminal profiles. The results of these studies demonstrate the unreliability of anecdotal evaluations and highlight the weakness of such an argument.

Key Words: Criminal profiles; anecdotal evaluations; accuracy.

Introduction

Despite the renown and apparent popularity of criminal profiling, particularly in law enforcement circles, it comes as something of a surprise that empirically robust evidence to support the merits of the technique has, until

*The following three chapters of this book will discuss a number of studies evaluating various aspects of criminal profiles and the practice of constructing a criminal profile. Incumbent to these studies are the use of statistical techniques to test and identify patterns and differences in the data. Any reader unfamiliar with such techniques may refer to Appendix A of this book, in which the elementary principles underpinning such methods are explained to assist in better understanding the subsequent chapters.

From: *Criminal Profiling: Principles and Practice*
By: R. N. Kocsis © Humana Press Inc., Totowa, NJ

quite recently, been remarkably scarce *(1)*. The studies discussed in Chapter 3 have endeavored to progress our scientific understanding of the comparative accuracy and requisite skills associated with the accurate construction of a criminal profile. Before considering the research findings canvassed in those chapters, however, it is important to question why, in the absence of scientifically rigorous material (the norm for virtually all other professional disciplines), the technique of criminal profiling has continued to prosper.

In one study by the author *(2)*, it was suggested that any combination of three possible factors might be operating to create this circumstance. The first factor involves the predominantly favorable, albeit sometimes fanciful, media glamorization that the technique enjoys *(3–5)*. On an intuitive level, fictional portrayals of criminal profiling may serve to fuel the impression of the merit and accuracy of the practice in assisting investigators. The second factor relates to the general environment in which criminal profiles are frequently used: criminal investigations, conducted by law enforcement agencies that typically feature comparatively insular authoritarian cultures *(6–14)*. Within such an environment, the technique of criminal profiling may not be exposed to the same degree of independent critical scrutiny that is characteristic of other scientifically constituted disciplines that feature considerable transparency and evaluation of internally adopted practices *(15,16)*. The third and arguably most pertinent factor in the context of this chapter relates to a circumstantial argument at times put forward by expert profilers when seeking to justify their practices *(17,18)*. This argument is described by the author *(2)* as the operational utilitarian argument, and is somewhat circular in what it posits. That is, if criminal profiles were not regarded as being useful, investigators such as police would simply not continue to use them. Accordingly, because police officers continue to use the services of expert profilers this circumstance serves as evidence attesting to the presumed merit and accuracy of the criminal profiles. In essence, the tenet underpinning the operational utilitarian argument is simply a variation of the old English proverb "the proof is in the pudding." That is, the accuracy of criminal profiles can be inferred by the circumstance of their continued use. Positive results, it seems, must be occurring because police officers continue to use criminal profiles to aid their investigations, and therefore the profiles must be accurate.

Despite the intuitive logic of such an argument, it has previously escaped empirical testing. Additionally, such an argument does not represent a direct and objective measure of the accuracy of a criminal profile. Instead, it is at best an indirect and inferred measure based on the perceived accuracy of the criminal profiles by users of them. That is, police officers perceive criminal profiles to be useful in the course of their investigations and consequently continue to use them. This circumstance is then taken as equating with evidence of the accuracy of a criminal profile.

One central premise underpinning the operational utilitarian argument is that the perceptions of police officers regarding the accuracy of a criminal profile are reliable. However, should these anecdotal evaluations be found to be unreliable in some respect, such as, for example, being subject to some extraneous influence or even bias, then the validity of the operational utilitarian argument would be seriously undermined. This question surrounding the reliability of anecdotal evaluations of criminal profiles is extremely pertinent when one considers the extensive history of psychological research that has consistently highlighted the unreliability of human perceptions in a wide variety of contexts *(19–21)*. Consequently, a series of studies were undertaken to investigate the reliability of such anecdotal evaluations. These studies sought to critically examine the validity of the operational utilitarian argument that has been relied on as evidence in support of the accuracy of criminal profiles for many decades.

*Evaluations of Criminal Profiles by Police Officers**

As previously explained, the underlying premise of the operational utilitarian argument is its reliance on anecdotal evaluations of criminal profiles. Accordingly, to test the validity of this argument one needs to examine the reliability of police officers' perceptions of a criminal profile. Consequently, a study was devised whereby a sample of police officers were presented with a criminal profile and asked to evaluate it on a quantifiable scale that could then be subjected to critical analysis *(22)*.

The first step in conducting this study involved obtaining 59 serving police officers who participated as the surveyed individuals for the study. The design of this study essentially involved providing the police officers with a survey that asked four questions concerning their evaluations of a criminal profile that accompanied the survey form. To explore the reliability of their evaluations and thus the possibility of some form of bias in their perceptions, some experimental variations (which are discussed next) were also incorporated into the study.

---

*The descriptions of the three studies canvassed throughout this chapter represent abridged summaries of the studies undertaken. Details inherent to each of these studies have been omitted to facilitate their easy comprehension in this book. Readers interested in this particular topic should consult the original manuscripts describing the studies in full *(22,23,27)*.

All of the survey forms started with the same cover page describing in general terms what criminal profiling is and how it is used in criminal investigations. Following this cover page, the survey forms provided some details concerning an actual murder. The description of this murder only provided a moderate amount of information and its purpose was to simply provide some background information regarding the nature of the survey for the police officers. A criminal profile followed this description of the murder. The survey form indicated that this profile was written by an individual who had been consulted by police officers to assist with their investigation into the aforementioned murder.

At this juncture, however, two important features were incorporated into the survey forms. The first feature related to the label that was provided to describe the author of the criminal profile. Although the survey forms indicated that the profile had been provided to assist the investigation, the identity of the author was deliberately altered among the different versions of the survey form. In half of the survey forms the criminal profile was labeled as written by a "professional profiler," whereas in the other half the identical profile was labeled as written by "someone the investigator consulted," thus providing a less descriptive label concerning the author. All of the survey forms requested that the criminal profile be carefully examined and four questions answered relating to its perceived merit. Aside from this variation concerning the identity of the author of the criminal profile, all of the survey forms contained the identical introductory material and asked the same four questions.

All four questions on the survey forms were measured on a 7-point scale in which 1 represented a low value rating, 4 an average rating, and 7 a very high rating. The first three questions all related to aspects of the perceived usefulness of the criminal profile. The first question asked for an evaluation of the perceived coherence of the criminal profile with respect to how well the ideas appeared to be presented. The second question inquired about the degree of specificity of the criminal profile with respect to how specific or vague the supplied information appeared. The third question inquired about the individuation of a suspect from the profile by asking for some estimation of how likely participants believed that the information contained in the profile would potentially help in narrowing a list of suspects. Following these three questions, a final separate section of the survey form was presented to the police officers. This section asked participants to rate the accuracy of the criminal profile. However, in this particular section of the survey an actual description of the apprehended murderer was also provided in the survey form. Consequently, when the police officers were making their evaluation of the accuracy of the profile they were undertaking a side-by-side comparison between the predictions constituting the criminal profile and the characteristics of the apprehended offender.

As previously mentioned, this study incorporated two special features. The first related to varying the listed identity of the author of the criminal profile. The second feature, however, was more aligned to strengthening the design of the study. One potential criticism of the study, as described thus far, might be that the obtained results could simply be an artifact of the particular criminal profile that was the subject of the experiment. That is, different results might be obtained by the use of a different criminal profile. To cater for this contingency, three different versions of the survey form that each contained one of three different criminal profiles was used. Each of the three versions of the survey consisted of one of two alternative conditions—one that listed the author of the criminal profile as the professional profiler and the other with the nondescript label of someone the investigator consulted. Consequently, this study featured six different versions of the survey form, one of which was randomly administered and completed by each of the 59 police officers. Their responses on the survey forms were scored together for each of the six respective versions and statistically analyzed for any differences in the mean scores for each different version of the survey.

As previously indicated, the purpose of this study was to test the reliability of police officers' anecdotal evaluations of a criminal profile and in the context of the design of this study it aimed to investigate whether the perceived merits of a criminal profile were affected by the labeled identity of the author.

The results of the analysis summarized in Table 2.1 indicate that when a criminal profile was simply labeled as authored by a professional profiler, it was consistently perceived to be more accurate than when the identical material was presented under the nondescript (i.e., anonymous) author label. Although the author label was found to influence the police officers' evaluation of the accuracy of a criminal profile, it did not, however, appear to affect their perceptions concerning its utility. Namely, the three measures related to coherence, specificity, or individuation.

Consequently, the findings of this study highlight the unreliability of anecdotal evaluations because some form of bias was found to be operating in the evaluation of the accuracy of a criminal profile by the sampled police officers.

Believing Is Seeing?

Although the previous study demonstrated that perceptions regarding the accuracy of a criminal profile appear to be influenced by the identity of its

Table 2.1
Police Perceptions of Criminal Profiles as a Function of the Labeled Identity of the Author Assigned to the Criminal Profile

	Author labels		
Profile measures	Anonymous ($n = 33$)	Profiler ($n = 26$)	
Coherence	No significant difference	No significant difference	
Specificity	No significant difference	No significant difference	
Individuation	No significant difference	No significant difference	
Accuracy	3.21	3.98	Significant differnce $F(1, 53) = 4.84, p < 0.05$

author, the study did not explore in any substantive capacity why this occurred. Accordingly, a second study was undertaken in an effort to understand the factors that may account for the observed bias in the previously surveyed police officers *(23)*.

Two theories were proposed by way of possible explanation. One theory related to the possibility of some intrinsic feature inherent to the police officers that may have accounted for their bias. For many decades, legal and criminological scholars have observed the strong collegiate sense of loyalty often present among members of policing organizations *(6–14)*. With these cultural loyalties in mind, perhaps the surveyed police officers identified the author title of professional profiler as someone affiliated with their organizational culture and thus were reluctant to assign an unfavorable rating to the work of a perceived colleague. The police officers may have, for example, objectively assessed the features of a criminal profile associated with its coherence, specificity, or individuation. However, the accuracy of the criminal profile may have been considered something directly reflective of a colleague's abilities. Consequently, this feature may have been judged more favorably when labeled as authored by a perceived colleague; thus the bias in evaluating the accuracy of the criminal profile.

The other theory offered to account for the bias relates to the confidence or belief that the sampled police officers may have held about criminal profiling. A number of studies in the social sciences have explored a phenomenon referred to as the Barnum effect, which accounts for the proclivities people demonstrate when interpreting ambiguous statements *(24)*. Researchers exploring the operation of the Barnum effect have observed that ambiguous material is often interpreted positively when there is some favorable link to the subject. For example, a study by Snyder and Newburg *(25)* found that people were more willing to accept ambiguous but positive descriptions about themselves than they were ambiguous but negative descriptions. Other research concerning the Barnum effect involved a study by Alison, Smith, and Morgan *(26)* that demonstrated that police officers had difficulty in discerning the amounts of valid information contained in a genuine, as opposed to fictitious, criminal profile. In view of such studies, perhaps the police officer's belief in profiling was encouraged when it was observed that the profile was authored by a professional profiler and thus evaluated it more favorably.

The objective of the second study was to investigate the plausibility of these two theories in accounting for the bias demonstrated by police officers in the previous study. Assuming that the bias was related to some intrinsic feature, such as the organizational culture of police, this bias then would presumably not be present in people external to policing. An initial test of this theory would simply involve repeating the previous study but with a sample of individuals who were not associated with policing. The second theory, however, operates on the existence of some conceptual relationship between a person's level of belief and their perceptions of a profile. If there were some basis to this theory, then variations in the levels of belief different people hold should be observable in their corresponding evaluation of a criminal profile.

Consequently, the design of this second study involved replicating the procedures used in the previous study with some additional measures. As previously stated, the theory concerning the cultural loyalty of police officers would involve a replication of the previous study but with individuals not subject to such cultural influences. Accordingly, the core components of the previous survey form were again administered, but this time to a sample of 353 university freshmen who were not associated with any police organization.

Testing the belief theory, however, required further adjustment to the previously administered survey. Namely, the inclusion of a measure that attempts to gauge a person's reported degree of belief in criminal profiling, which could be concurrently compared with their evaluation of the accuracy of a criminal profile. Akin to the scales described in the previous study, another five questions were created that asked a respondent to rate their belief in whether a criminal profile could effectively predict certain characteristics. For example, one question asked, "Do you believe profiles can accurately predict the gender of an unknown offender? Please rate your confidence on a scale from 1 to 7, where 1 = *No, probably incorrect* and 7 = *Yes, probably correct*." By tallying the ratings of these five questions, a quantitative score could be obtained that reflected a respondent's degree of belief in criminal profiling.

As previously mentioned, the belief theory presupposes the existence of some conceptual relationship between the level of belief a person possesses and the perceptions of an individual regarding a criminal profile. If this concept were valid, then variations in the level of a person's belief would presumably be observable in the evaluations made by them concerning a criminal profile. To test this idea, three different cover pages were developed for each of the survey forms. One of the cover pages described criminal profiling in purely favorable, positive terms. The purpose of this cover page was to convey a sense of confidence in criminal profiling and thus encourage the person's level of belief. A second version of the cover page described criminal profiling in highly unfavorable, negative terms. The purpose of this cover page was to promote disbelief and skepticism in criminal profiling. Finally, the third cover page was created to serve as a neutral or control condition. This version of the cover page simply sought to provide an equivalent reading exercise to the other two cover pages and contained information totally unrelated to criminal profiling. This acted as a conceptual benchmark between the two polarities of positive and negative beliefs in criminal profiling.

The survey forms for this study were thus compiled to have three separate belief conditions. One belief condition deliberately attempted to bolster belief in profiling (i.e., positive), another served as a control condition (i.e., neutral), and the third sought to undermine an individual's level of belief in profiling (i.e., negative). Attached to each of these three cover pages were the five questions developed to measure an individual's reported level of belief. The survey form instructed the reader to answer these five questions immediately after reading the cover page. Once an individual had finished responding to the five questions concerning their belief in profiling the remainder of the survey form was akin to the one used in the first study *(22)* with one exception.

In the previous study, the accuracy of the criminal profile was evaluated by a side-by-side comparison with the details of the offender revealed to the participants at the very end of the survey on a separate form. In the present study, an extra measure was incorporated in an effort to assess the perceived accuracy of the criminal profile without the benefit of the description of the offender. This was accomplished by simply adding another question that asked the participant to evaluate the accuracy of the criminal profile immediately after the three questions that asked about the utility of the profile (i.e., coherence, specificity, and individuation). Then, as described in the previous study *(22)*, the question relating to accuracy was again asked, but in a totally separate section of the survey form where a description of the offender was also provided. Thus, the question that requested an evaluation without the benefit of a description of the offender simulated the circumstance of an on-going investigation in which the identity of the offender is unknown, whereas the side-by-side comparison simulated an evaluation subsequent to the apprehension of the offender.

Table 2.2
Relationships Between Levels of Reported Belief and Profile Evaluations

Profile measures	Correlation value	Significance (p)	
Coherence	0.32	<0.001	Significant incremental relationship
Specificity	0.13	0.013	Significant incremental relationship
Individuation	0.30	<0.001	Significant incremental relationship
Estimated accuracy	0.47	<0.001	Significant incremental relationship
Compared accuracy	0.16	0.002	Significant incremental relationship

Sample size ($N = 353$). Significance level (i.e., $\alpha = 0.05$).

Significant positive relationships found to exist between an individual's level of belief and his or her rating on all of the profile evaluation measures.

Consequently, the survey instrument in this second study was modified to reflect three different versions based on the differing belief condition (i.e., positive, negative, and neutral). Each of these three belief conditions contained six separate subconditions (akin to the first study) reflective of the three different criminal profiles with alternating author titles. Accordingly, in this second study, 18 different versions of the survey form (i.e., 3 × 6) were created. One of these 18 possible versions of the survey form was then randomly given to each of the 353 university freshmen (i.e., students).

Once again, the responses to these surveys were tallied for each of the respective versions and subjected to statistical analysis to investigate whether any differences or patterns could be discerned from the derived data (Table 2.2).

The results of this analysis were revealing in what they indicated about the proposed theories. First, the students did not demonstrate any significant differences in their evaluations based on the author label of the criminal profiles. This finding differs from the previous study *(22)* in which the police officers consistently perceived a criminal profile to be more accurate when labeled as having been written by a professional profiler. Consequently, this result lends some tentative support to the contention that the bias observed in the previous study may indeed be related to some intrinsic feature of the previously sampled police officers.

Equally revealing, however, were the results concerning the relationship between an individual's reported level of belief in criminal profiling and their evaluations of a criminal profile. As summarized in Table 2.2, significant incremental relationships (i.e., statistical correlations) were found to exist between the reported level of belief an individual held and their evaluations of a criminal profile on all of the measures incorporated in this study. Thus, the more an individual believed in criminal profiling, the more favorably they evaluated a criminal profile, be it in the coherence, individuation, specificity, or accuracy stakes. This finding suggests that the famous adage "seeing is believing" appears to operate in reverse with respect to criminal profiles. That is, simply believing in criminal profiling is quite likely to result in seeing a criminal profile more favorably. Perhaps the most alarming aspect of this phenomenon is that one of the strongest manifestations of this relationship occurs when evaluating the accuracy of a criminal profile (i.e., the estimated accuracy of a profile).

Beliefs and the Content of Criminal Profiles

Although the second study provided some evidence for the existence of a relationship between an individual's level of belief in criminal profiling and the perceived merits of a profile, the study offered little insight into what components of information contained in a criminal profile might contribute to this phenomenon. Consequently, a third study was undertaken to specifically investigate this issue as well as to test the reliability of the previous findings.

Once again, the overall design of this third study closely followed that of its predecessor *(23)*. Virtually all components of the survey form previously described for the second study were reproduced. Eighteen different versions of the survey form were used, comprised of the three belief conditions (i.e., cover pages with information describing profiling in either a positive, negative, or neutral context followed by the questions to rate their belief in criminal profiling). Each of the three belief conditions contained six different subversions of the survey form using one of the three different criminal profiles with the author label being alternated (i.e., between either professional profiler or someone the investigator consulted) on each of the three profiles. Once again, another sample of 353 university freshmen were recruited to participate in this study.*

The only change in design to this third study was the replacement of the three questions that asked participants to evaluate the criminal profile in terms of its perceived individuation, specificity, and coherence. In place of these

*It should be noted that by pure coincidence the final number of people who completed the survey form in this third study was identical to that of the previous study (i.e., 353). Thus, a total of 706 people were surveyed in conducting these two separate studies.

questions were 39 very short questions that asked the respondent to indicate whether the profile provided some description of a nominated characteristic of the likely offender.* A few examples of these questions included, "Does the criminal profile describe the offender's likely build?" (Y/N) or "Does the criminal profile describe any prior relationship between the victim and the offender?" (Y/N).

Consequently, these questions measured the type and amount of information perceived to be in a criminal profile. To maximize the interpretability of the data derived from these 39 questions, three categories were developed indicative of the type of information they broadly represented. Thus, 8 of the questions related to whether the criminal profile described some type of physical feature of the likely offender and dealt with physical descriptors of the offender, such as age and gender. Another 16 of the questions related to whether the profile described some aspect of the offender's background history and other historical aspects, such as the offender's level of education or vocational history. The remaining 15 questions asked whether the profile described any specific crime behaviors and referred to information pertaining to the likely actions and events surrounding the commission of the offense.

Akin to the procedures of the previous study, one of the 18 different versions of the survey form was randomly administered to the sampled university freshmen. The scores on each of the survey forms were tallied together in each of the respective conditions and then subjected to various forms of statistical analyses to discern whether any differences or patterns emerged from the data (Table 2.3).

Similar to the findings of the second study, no differences were found among the freshmen regarding the perceived merit of a criminal profile based on the labeled identity of the author. This result provides further evidence to suggest that the bias observed in the first study may indeed be related to some intrinsic feature of the previously sampled police officers.

As summarized in Table 2.3, an incremental relationship was again found between the level of belief in criminal profiling and the perceptions of the accuracy of a criminal profile. However, the results of this third study also indicated that an incremental relationship existed between an individual's level of belief and the amount of information related to background history and crime behaviors perceived to be contained in a criminal profile. This relationship, however, was not found to exist with respect to perceptions of the physical

*These 39 questions were structured in a dichotomous format so that the answer to each question was either a "yes" or "no." The 39 questions reflecting information typically contained in a criminal profile originated from another study that is discussed in Chapter 4 *(28)*.

Table 2.3
Relationships Between Levels of Reported "Belief" and Perceptions of Content and Accuracy in Criminal Profiles

Profile measures	Correlation value	Significance (p)	
Background history (16 questions)	0.13	0.014	Significant incremental relationship
Crime behaviors (15 questions)	0.19	<0.001	Significant incremental relationship
Physical features (8 questions)	0.038	0.483	No relationship
Estimated accuracy	0.48	<0.001	Significant incremental relationship
Compared accuracy	0.313	<0.001	Significant incremental relationship

Sample size ($N = 353$). Significance level (i.e., $\alpha = 0.05$).

characteristics of the offender. Consequently, this third study demonstrates that in addition to the existence of an incremental relationship between belief and perceived accuracy, the higher the level of belief, the greater the amount of information that will be perceived to be present in a criminal profile pertaining to background history and crime behaviors.

Conclusion

The findings of the three studies discussed in this chapter highlight the unreliability of anecdotal evaluations of criminal profiles and thus clearly challenge the validity of the operational utilitarian argument. In contrast to the premise of the argument, these studies suggest that police officers may erroneously perceive greater accuracy in a criminal profile.

Perhaps even more intriguing are the indications of a relationship existing between the level of belief an individual possesses in criminal profiling and their corresponding evaluation of a criminal profile. As outlined at the start of this chapter, the practice of criminal profiling has enjoyed predominantly favorable popular culture depictions over the past decades *(3–5)*. Therefore, it needs to be questioned to what extent, such depictions may have subconsciously influenced the levels of belief that police officers and others in the community may have about profiling and the extent to which such impressions influence their evaluations concerning the accuracy of a criminal profile. It could be that the operational utilitarian argument may, in fact, be little more than the manifestation of a vicious illusionary cycle. That is, popular culture representations and anecdotal testimonials may artificially elevate people's belief in the capabilities of profiling. These elevated beliefs may in turn lead to misconceptions concerning the accuracy and merit of criminal profiles. Such misconceptions may then in turn sponsor the continued use of profiling and perhaps lead to even more favorable media coverage and testimonials: thus the cycle continues.

No doubt the findings of these studies are likely to prove confronting to expert profilers who seek to justify their practices with any sort of operational utilitarian argument. Unfortunately, anecdotal examples and testimonials as justification for the validity of criminal profiles may amount to little more than smoke and mirrors. These studies illustrate how imperative it is that the merits of criminal profiles be assessed through independent scientifically controlled studies.

References

1. Oleson, J.C. (1996). Psychological profiling: Does it actually work? Forensic Update, 46, 11–14.
2. Kocsis, R.N. (2003). Criminal psychological profiling: Validities and abilities? International Journal of Offender Therapy and Comparative Criminology, 47(2), 126–144.
3. Harris, T. (1985). The red dragon. New York: Heineman.
4. Harris, T. (1986). The silence of the lambs. New York: Heineman.
5. Harris, T. (1999). Hannibal. New York: Heineman.
6. Chan, J.B.L. (1996). Changing police culture. British Journal of Criminology, 36(1), 109–134.
7. Chan, J.B.L. (1997). Changing police culture: Policing a multicultural society. Cambridge: Cambridge University Press.
8. DeMaria, W. (1999). Deadly disclosures. Adelaide: Wakefield Press.
9. Dempster, Q. (1997). Whistleblowers. Sydney: ABC Books.
10. Finnane, M. (1995). From police force to police service? Aspects of the recent history of the New South Wales Police. Unpublished manuscript prepared for the Wood Royal Commission into the New South Wales Police Service.
11. Fitzgerald, R. (1989). Report of a commission of inquiry pursuant to orders in council: Commission of inquiry into possible illegal activities and associated police misconduct. Brisbane: Queensland Government Press.
12. Lusher, R. (1981). Report of the commission of inquiry into the New South Wales Police administration. Sydney: NSW Government Printer.
13. Miethe, T.D. (1999). Whistleblowing at work: Tough choices in exposing fraud, waste and abuse on the job. Boulder: Westview Press.
14. Wood, J.R.T. (1997). Royal commission into the New South Wales Police Service: Final report. Sydney: NSW Government Printer.
15. Kocsis, R.N. and Coleman, S. (2000). The unexplored ethics of criminal psychological profiling, In: Godwin, M.G., ed. Criminal psychology and forensic technology: A collaborative approach to effective profiling. New York: CRC Press, pp. 323–338.

16. Kocsis, R.N. and Palermo, G.B. (2005). Ten major problems with criminal profiling. American Journal of Forensic Psychiatry, 26(2), 45–67.
17. Jeffers, H.P. (1992). Profiles in evil. London: Warner Bros.
18. US House of Representative (1990). U.S.S. Iowa tragedy: An investigative failure: Report of the investigations subcommittee and the defense policy panel of the committee on armed services. Washington, DC: Author.
19. Hamilton, D.L. and Zanna, M.P. (1972). Differential weighting of favorable attributes in impressions of personality. Journal of Experimental Research in Personality, 6, 204–212.
20. Merton, R. (1948). The self-fulfilling prophecy. Antioch Review, 8, 193–210.
21. Heider, F. (1958). The psychology of interpersonal relations. New York: Wiley.
22. Kocsis, R.N. and Hayes, A.F. (2004). Believing is seeing? Investigating the perceived accuracy of criminal psychological profiles. International Journal of Offender Therapy and Comparative Criminology, 48(2), 149–160.
23. Kocsis, R.N. and Heller, G.Z. (2004) Believing is seeing—II. Beliefs and perceptions of criminal psychological profiles. International Journal of Offender Therapy and Comparative Criminology, 48(3), 313–329.
24. Dickson, D.H. and Kelly, I.W. (1985). The 'Barnum effect' in personality assessment: A review of the literature. Psychological Reports, 57, 367–382.
25. Snyder, C.R. and Newburg, C.L. (1981). The Barnum effect in a group setting. J Pers Assess, 45, 622–629.
26. Alison, L.J., Smith, M.D., and Morgan, K. (2003). Interpreting the accuracy of offender profiles. Psychology, Crime and Law, 9(2), 185–195.
27. Kocsis, R.N. and Middledorp, J.T. (2004) Believing is Seeing—III. Perceptions of content in criminal psychological profiles. International Journal of Offender Therapy and Comparative Criminology, 48(4), 477–494.
28. Kocsis, R.N. (2003). An empirical assessment of content in criminal psychological profiles. International Journal of Offender Therapy and Comparative Criminology, 47(1), 38–47.

Chapter 3

Rhetoric vs Reality

Investigating the Skills and Accuracy of Criminal Profiling

Summary

Through a series of empirical studies, the accuracy of criminal profiles as constructed by expert profilers and numerous other skill-based groups are assessed in this chapter. The findings of these studies provide some tentative evidence to suggest that criminal profiles constructed by expert profilers have a comparatively higher degree of accuracy in their predictions. These studies, however, also suggest that the skill base most likely to be aligned with the proficient construction of a criminal profile primarily relate to an individual's capacity to engage in logical and objective reasoning. These findings challenge the previously held, yet empirically untested, view that skills inherent to the proficient construction of a criminal profile are sourced in investigative experience.

Key Words: Criminal profiles; accuracy; skills; logical and objective reasoning.

Introduction

Arguably, the most fundamental question underpinning criminal profiling is whether the technique actually works, or more specifically, whether the predictions of profilers in describing the characteristics of an unknown offender are accurate. Despite the seemingly obvious nature of this question, rigorous empirical data to answer it has been in short supply. This observation, however, should not be interpreted as implying that the development of criminal profiling has occurred within a total vacuum. On the contrary, much material in the form of anecdotal accounts attesting to the merits of criminal profiles has been promulgated in support of their accuracy. Unfortunately,

From: *Criminal Profiling: Principles and Practice*
By: R. N. Kocsis © Humana Press Inc., Totowa, NJ

these anecdotal examples seldom appear in publications that are subject to the rigors of independent scientific review. Instead, they frequently originate from true crime novels often co-authored by retired profilers *(1–3)*. Furthermore, although such anecdotal examples may illustrate the application of a criminal profile, the various studies canvassed in the previous chapter clearly indicate that these accounts cannot be relied on as equating with evidence in support of the scientific veracity of profiling as a valid technique *(4–6)*.

Another source of material that is sometimes offered as evidence for the validity of profiling are user satisfaction surveys *(7–9)*. Although these surveys are informative in reflecting the satisfaction investigators derive from the use of a criminal profile, it is important to appreciate that satisfaction with a service does not necessarily equate with its validity. Indeed, the studies of the previous chapter warn of the perils of making such inferences.

It is perhaps difficult to appreciate, but independent, empirically based, scientifically vetted evidence to test the accuracy of profilers and thus criminal profiling has, until quite recently, been surprisingly scarce *(10)*. Possibly the first piece of empirical evidence to consider the accuracy of criminal profiling emerged in one subcomponent of a study conducted by Pinizzotto and Finkel *(11)*. These researchers undertook a number of small experiments that were designed to examine differing aspects surrounding the practice of constructing a criminal profile, the most pertinent being an experiment that involved the construction of criminal profiles for two actual crimes. Possibly the most important feature to this experiment was that it empirically, and more significantly, objectively scored the profiles and thereby measured the accuracy of the predictions contained in them. The design of the experiment involved obtaining case materials compiled by a police investigation into a previously solved murder and rape case. Accompanying these materials was a small, multiple-choice questionnaire relating to the possible characteristics of the offender(s), such as age, gender, occupation, and so on. With these case materials and the accompanying questionnaire, a profiling simulation using an actual crime was developed. Given that the offenses were previously solved and the identity of the offender known by the researchers but withheld from the participants, the accuracy of their predictions could be reliably scored. That is, the multiple-choice questionnaire created a means by which the accuracy of the predictions could be objectively assessed. The questionnaire did not allow for any ambiguity and/or subjectivity in attempting to interpret the accuracy of predictions. Akin to most other tests that make use of multiple-choice questionnaires, the responses were structured in such a way that it was clearly determinable whether the prediction concerning some characteristic of the probable offender was right or wrong.

Following this design, Pinizzotto and Finkel *(11)* tested four small groups of participants on both the murder and rape case materials. These groups consisted of trained profilers, psychologists, detectives, and university students. The results of this experiment provided a comparative demonstration of the proficiency the differing groups exhibited in their capacity to accurately profile the characteristics of the unknown offender(s) in the murder and rape case. Based on their expertise and training, profilers were expected to surpass the other three groups. The results of this experiment, however, were a far cry from unequivocally endorsing the efforts of profilers. In profiling the perpetrator of the murder case, the profilers failed to surpass any of the other groups and ironically, their overall level of accuracy was found to be descriptively the lowest. However, in profiling the perpetrator of the rape case, the profilers indeed surpassed the other three groups in the level of accuracy they demonstrated in predicting the characteristics of the unknown rapist.

It was in recognition of the paucity of critical examination of criminal profiling beyond Pinizzotto and Finkel's *(11)* study that prompted the further investigation of the skills and accuracy inherent to the construction of criminal profiles.

Skills and Accuracy in Profiling: An Initial Examination

One of the most surprising findings of Pinizzotto and Finkel's *(11)* experiment was the poor performance of the profilers in predicting the characteristics of the unknown murderer despite criminal profiling often being presented as most suitable to crimes of murder *(1,3,12,13)*. Consequently, it was determined that a larger, dedicated study* should be undertaken that examined the proficiency of expert profilers in their assessment of a murder.

Beyond simply measuring the proficiency of profilers, however, it was also considered valuable to undertake some empirically driven analysis of the constituent skills that may underpin an individual's capacity to generate an accurate profile. Once again, empirically based consideration of this issue was remarkably scarce with the only literature at that time provided by a chapter by Hazelwood et al. *(14)*, which proposed a number of attributes as essential for the effective construction of a criminal profile. Chief among these attributes was an appreciation of the criminal mind, intuition, investigative experience, and logical and objective reasoning.

---

*It should be remembered that the described experiment by Pinizzotto and Finkel *(11)* only represented one small subcomponent of their study.

Consequently, a study was undertaken that built on the design of Pinizzotto and Finkel's *(11)* experiment by developing an experiment whereby participants' abilities in profiling the characteristics of an unknown murderer could be tested via an objective and quantifiable multiple-choice questionnaire* *(15)*. The very first step in undertaking this study involved obtaining the case materials as compiled by a police investigation into a previously solved murder. These materials featured such things as officer and witness statements, forensic reports, schematic diagrams, and photographs of the crime scenes just before the perpetrator of the murder was actually apprehended. These case materials were assembled and effectively represented the information available to police personnel concerning the murder just before the murderer had been identified. Accompanying these case materials was a multiple-choice questionnaire in which respondents were asked to provide their predictions concerning the characteristics of the offender via the multiple-choice options. As mentioned previously, the experiment by Pinizzotto and Finkel *(11)* was only a small subcomponent of their overall study and thus their multiple-choice questionnaire to survey possible offender characteristics consisted of a relatively small number of questions. To improve on this limited measure, a much larger multiple-choice questionnaire was developed that surveyed a broader scope of offender characteristics likely to be featured in a criminal profile. The questionnaire consisted of 33 distinct questions that surveyed characteristics of the unknown offender, such as their physical features; cognitive processes associated with the commission of the murder; behaviors before, during, and after the murder; and their general history and habits. As the murder had been solved, the questionnaire was then given to the detective who apprehended the offender in the case. A set of model answers to the questionnaire was developed by engaging the detective, who was intimately familiar with the case and the characteristics of the murderer. Using these model answers, copies of the questionnaire completed by other participants who were unaware of the identity of the offender could then be objectively scored for accuracy.

The next step in this study involved testing various skill-based groups and comparing their performance in terms of the level of accuracy they could then respectively achieve in profiling the characteristics of the unknown murderer based on examination of the case materials. As the key feature of this study was to examine the capabilities of profilers (and thereby the efficacy of

*For brevity and ease of comprehension, only an abridged summation of this and all subsequent studies is discussed in this book.

profiling), a sample of five expert profilers was obtained. These individuals were all recognized as skilled professionals in the construction of criminal profiles and had each previously been consulted by law enforcement agencies to assist with an investigation by constructing a criminal profile. In addition to the profilers, it was important to examine the capabilities of various other individuals who could then serve as points of comparison for the performance of the expert profilers. However, as previously mentioned, it was considered useful to be able to identify some skill base inherent to each of these groups because it may be reflective of their level of performance in accurately predicting the characteristics of the unknown murderer. The identification of any skills may account for a sample group's proficiency in profiling. The first skill considered was an appreciation of the criminal mind. Although Hazelwood et al. *(14)* suggest that this skill does not necessarily need to be learned by formal education, they do nonetheless acknowledge that a background in behavioral sciences, such as psychology and psychological skills, is clearly beneficial. Consequently, to operationalize such skill into a group of participants that were readily distinguishable and representative of psychological skills, a sample of 30 psychologists was obtained.

In the opinion of Hazelwood et al., "No amount of education can replicate the experience of having investigated crimes" (*14*, p. 119), thus investigative experience is proposed by these authors as quintessential for the proficient construction of a criminal profile. Although a number of professions can lay claim to investigative experience, the most readily apparent group (and arguably the group Hazelwood et al. envisaged) that could be expected to demonstrate it are experienced police officers. Thus, a sample of 35 police officers was also recruited. In addition to investigative experience, Hazelwood et al. *(14)* also indicate that effective profilers are characterized by their capacity for logical and objective reasoning and thus are not easily diverted by personal feelings concerning the crime under consideration. To address this skill dimension, a sample of 30 science students were recruited who did not possess any training or experience in psychology or criminal investigation but had, through their studies in science, been trained to set aside personal impressions in the rational analysis of information. Beyond investigative experience or logical and objective reasoning, Hazelwood et al. *(14)* also identified the psychic-like faculty of intuition as another constituent skill inherent to proficient profiling. Although some researchers *(16)* have attempted to discount the almost mystical portrayal of profilers, Hazelwood et al. nonetheless nominate intuition as a requisite skill for profiling. Accordingly, to gain some impression of this factor 20 professional psychics—individuals reliant on their intuitive abilities—were also recruited.

Consequently, this study involved groups of profilers, psychologists, police officers, science students, and psychics undertaking the criminal profiling exercise for the previously described murder case *(15)*. It was hoped that the assembly of such survey participants would provide some insight into their respective proficiency in accurately profiling the characteristics of the murderer as well as the relative importance of the skills inherent to each of the groups.

Additionally, one final group was also included. Criticism concerning criminal profiling has often centered around the usefulness of the information profiles contain. For example, Godwin *(17)* likened the information contained in criminal profiles to that attainable from the local bartender. Although colloquial in expression, Godwin *(17)* is justified in questioning the value of the information contained in criminal profiles. Are the predictions of profilers, or any other skill-based group for that matter, capable of making predictions better than what could be achieved through stereotypical conceptions of the typical offender, or simply by guessing (i.e., luck)? To investigate this idea, a group of 23 economics students was also recruited to participate in the study. These students were selected principally on the basis that they did not possess any identifiable skill basis related to any of the other recruited groups. These economic students, however, were not given any of the case material concerning the murder to be profiled but were simply provided with the 33-item multiple-choice questionnaire. This group was then asked to complete the questionnaire by nominating what they believed to be the characteristics of the typical murderer. By this procedure, some impression could be gained about the relative score on the questionnaire an individual could achieve by simply guessing or using stereotypical notions of what the characteristics of the typical murderer may be. Thus, this group can be viewed as a control condition for comparison with the performance of the other tested groups.

Thus, all participants completed this profiling exercise and their responses were scored for accuracy using the model answers previously developed. All scores were then compiled for their respective groups and subjected to statistical analysis. The results of this analysis are summarized in Table 3.1.

As indicated in Table 3.1, the group that achieved the highest mean score and thus demonstrated the greatest comparative degree of accuracy in predicting the characteristics of the unknown murderer were the profilers. Following the profilers were the psychologists, then the science students, police officers, psychics, and finally the control condition of the economic students who responded to the questionnaire by relying on guesswork and stereotypical conceptions of a typical murderer. Although the differences in accuracy scores between the various groups are discernable, they should nonetheless be regarded as providing only tentative indications. There are two reasons for

Table 3.1
Mean Profile Accuracy Scores of Each of the Groups

	Profilers ($n = 5$)	Psychologists ($n = 30$)	Students ($n = 31$)	Police ($n = 35$)	Psychics ($n = 20$)	Control (no case material; $n = 23$)
Accuracy score	13.8^{a}	12.57^{b}	12.03^{c}	11.6^{d}	11.3	$9.78^{a,b,c,d}$

^{a,b,c,d}Statistically significant differences between groups are denoted by the same superscripted letter (e.g., *a* and *a*).

this caution. First, the number of sampled participants in some of the groups, most importantly the expert profilers, is quite small and thus the statistical representation of their number is limited. Second, although these numerical differences in the accuracy scores are descriptively visible, the number of statistically significant differences between the groups are limited.

What is perhaps more revealing from these results are the insights they offer concerning the constituent skills associated with proficient profiling. Based on the skill base represented by each of the groups (excluding the profilers), it seems apparent that skills associated with an understanding of human behavior, as denoted by the performance of the psychologists, seem to be the most closely aligned, in this study at least, with proficient profiling. The next most important skill appears to be a capacity for logical and objective analysis as denoted by the scores of the science students. Despite the emphasis Hazelwood et al. *(14)* appear to place on the skill of investigative experience in criminal profiling, the accuracy scores for the sampled police did not appear to support this notion when compared with the scores obtained by the other groups.

Possibly the most striking result to emerge from this study relates to the performance of the psychics and the input of intuition. As previously mentioned, the number of statistically significant differences between the accuracy scores of the various groups were limited. In this respect, the only statistically significant differences found in the accuracy scores were between each of the respective groups and the control condition—with the exception of the psychics, which indicates that each of the groups (i.e., profilers, psychologists, science students, and police officers) performed better in predicting the characteristics of the murderer than what could have been achieved through guesswork and/or relying on stereotypical notions of the typical murderer—as was the circumstance with the control group. However, the accuracy score of the sampled psychics was not found to be statistically different in terms of surpassing the score of the control group. Consequently, this indicates that the performance of the psychics in profiling the murderer was actually no better than what could have been achieved by simply guessing and suggests that the attribute of intuition is unlikely to play a meaningful role in the construction of an accurate criminal profile.

Investigative Experience and Criminal Profiling Revisited

Although the previous study provided some tentative indications for the abilities of profilers, it also highlighted the comparative differences in scores of the various groups and the constituent skills for profiling they each represented. Perhaps most notable was the relatively poor performance of the police officers, despite Hazelwood et al. *(14)* placing particular emphasis on investigative experience as possibly the quintessential skill for criminal profiling. Indeed, a number of profiler training programs, including that conducted by the FBI's Behavioral Science Unit, emphasize the importance of investigative experience by identifying seniority and accomplishment in policing as essential prerequisites for entry into their training programs *(1–3,18)*.

Given the stark contrast between this frequently promulgated view regarding the importance of investigative experience and the empirical evidence of the previous study, a more focused examination of these issues seemed warranted. Consequently, a second study was undertaken to specifically investigate this issue further *(19)*. It seems reasonable to assume from the views of Hazelwood et al. *(14)* that the relative importance of investigative experience would be dependent on the amount of such experience an individual possesses. The underlying notion appears to be that of an incremental relationship between an individual's amount of investigative experience and the degree of accuracy they are likely to demonstrate in profiling a violent crime. Simply put, individuals with greater amounts of investigative experience would be expected to be more competent in accurately profiling the perpetrator of a crime in comparison with individuals with lesser amounts or no investigative experience. To some extent, this notion is borne out by the recruitment practices of organizations, such as the FBI *(1–3,18)*.

Accordingly, one method of empirically testing investigative experience would simply involve repeating the previous study but focusing on surveying differing groups of people who could be distinguished by the amount of investigative experience they respectively possessed. Consequently, the identical survey instrument developed in the previous study *(15)* concerning the solved murder case and accompanying multiple-choice questionnaire was again used. However, in this second study differing groups of people distinguished by their respective levels of investigative experience were obtained to complete the survey.

Four separate groups of police personnel were recruited for this study. The first group was comprised of 12 detectives who worked within a specialized homicide unit and focused exclusively on the investigation of crimes of homicide, and specifically, murders. The second group was comprised of 31 senior detectives who, in addition to having served as general duty officers, each possessed a minimum of 10 years experience in criminal investigation as detectives. The third recruited group consisted of 19 trainee detectives. These were serving police officers who possessed at least 10 years experience as police officers undertaking general duties and were currently undergoing training to become detectives to specialize in criminal investigations.

The fourth group consisted of 50 police recruits. These participants were all undergoing training to become serving police officers. These individuals did not possess any prior experience as police officers but were interested in pursuing a career in policing and were very near the end of their training to commence active duty as a probationary (i.e., "rookie") officer.

Accordingly, these four groups represented a gradient of investigative experience. The homicide and senior detectives both possessed greater amounts of investigative experience; the trainee detective group was something of an intermediary, consisting of police officers with experience but not necessarily in criminal investigations; and the police recruits had very little experience beyond their basic training. Finally, to further contrast the input of investigative experience with people who did not possess any experience in law enforcement whatsoever, two further groups were recruited to participate in this second study. First, and akin to the previous study, a sample of 31 science students who possessed skills in logical and objective reasoning was obtained. Second, a control group was obtained consisting of 50 individuals who did not possess any particularly representative skills in comparison with these other groups and who were not provided with any case materials but instead completed the questionnaire by simply guessing and/or relying on stereotypical conceptions of a murderer.

Akin to the procedures of the previous study all of these groups were provided with the case materials and questionnaire (with the exception of the control group) and each endeavored to profile the characteristics of the murderer by answering the multiple-choice questions listed on the questionnaire. The responses on each of the questionnaires were then scored for accuracy. All scores were then compiled into their respective groups and subjected to statistical analysis (Table 3.2).

To make the results of the present study comparable with other research, the analysis of the present data was not only undertaken using the 33-item questionnaire of the previous study but also by using the equivalent questions that were used in Pinizzotto and Finkel's *(11)* study.* The analysis of the data using both of these measures yielded reasonably similar results, which are summarized in Table 3.2.

In stark contrast to the promulgated importance of investigative experience, the results of this study provide little support for this contention. Instead, a pattern emerges in the mean scores in which participants with less investi-

* It should be noted that this analysis, in using the analogous questions used by Pinizzotto and Finkel *(11)*, was also adopted in the original study *(15)* but, once again, for brevity are not canvassed in this chapter.

Table 3.2
Mean Profile Accuracy Scores Between Groups

	Homicide detectives ($n = 12$)	Senior detectives ($n = 31$)	Trainee detectives ($n = 19$)	Police recruits ($n = 50$)	Students ($n = 31$)	Control (no case material; $n = 50$)
Smaller measure (Pinizzotto and Finkel, 1990; *11*)	3.33^{d}	3.68^{b}	3.68	4.20^{c}	$4.58^{a,b,d}$	$3.22^{a,c}$
Total accuracy	9.92^{b}	11.58	11.84	11.78	$12.39^{a,b}$	10.64^{a}

^{a,b,c,d}Overall statistical differences are present between groups with specific pair-wise differences denoted by the same superscripted letter (e.g., *a* and *a*).

gative experience tend to demonstrate higher degrees of accuracy, whereas individuals with more investigative experience tend to achieve lower degrees of accuracy. Furthermore, the science students who possessed no investigative experience whatsoever actually surpassed the homicide and senior detectives* at a statistically significant level. These patterns are quite revealing because they are in stark contrast to Hazelwood et al.'s *(14)* contention concerning investigative experience. Clearly, if investigative experiences were indeed a quintessential skill, we would expect both of these groups of police officers to fair better in accurately profiling the murderer's characteristics.

Surprisingly, none of the police groups (with one exception†) irrespective of their level of investigative experience, demonstrated a significantly superior degree of proficiency in profiling the characteristics of the murderer beyond what could have been achieved by guessing and/or relying on stereotypical notions. That is, akin to the performance of the psychics in the previous study, the scores of the various police groups were not found to be different at a statistically significant level from that of the control group. The only group that was found to consistently surpass the control condition at a statistically significant level were, in fact, the science students.

In conclusion, the results of this second study were unable to support the contention concerning the importance, let alone the quintessential nature, of investigative experience as a requisite skill for accurately constructing a criminal profile.

Crime Modality, Investigative Specialization, and Criminal Profile Accuracy

The lack of support for the input of investigative experience in the previous study *(19)* was a finding of some consternation especially in light of the popularity of notions, such as those of Hazelwood et al. *(14)*. Indeed, some argument remained as to whether the previous two studies had adequately explored all dimensions of what might be encapsulated by the skill of investigative experience. For example, the previous study considered investigative experience primarily in quantitative terms by the number of years of experi-

* It should be clarified that statistically significant differences between senior detectives and students were only found in the smaller measure.

† This one exception being the police recruits when assessed using the smaller measure of questions analogous to from Pinizzotto and Finkel's *(11)* study. However, this standard of performance was not sustained when compared using the full measure of all 33 questionnaire items.

ence the differing groups possessed in law enforcement. Perhaps, however, implicit in Hazelwood et al.'s *(14)* proposition concerning investigative experience was a qualitative dimension. That is, it is not purely the number of years of experience *per se* in law enforcement or even in investigating crimes, but rather, experience in investigating the types of crime that are relevant to criminal profiling or at least relevant to profiling the crime in question. Although this qualitative dimension is not articulated in Hazelwood et al.'s *(14)* description of investigative experience, it does nonetheless represent a reasonable and plausible factor. Merely because a police officer possesses many years of experience in the investigation of armed robberies, for example, does not necessarily mean that that the same officer would necessarily possess the kind of investigative experience suitable for the profiling of a murder. Rather, for the profiling of a murder, experience in the investigation of murder would be pertinent. Arguably, therefore, various types of investigative experience might exist that do not necessarily transpose into differing contexts. Consequently, it is important to match the appropriate type of investigative experience with the appropriate type of crime being profiled. In some limited capacity, this qualitative dimension to investigative experience had already received some consideration in the previous study with the inclusion of the homicide squad detectives who exclusively worked in the investigation of homicide. Although the homicide squad detectives performed relatively poorly in the previous study, a separate study focusing on this qualitative aspect seemed to be warranted, given the nature of the results.

Consequently, a third study was undertaken that specifically considered this qualitative dimension of investigative experience with two added variations. The first of these variations considered the influence crime modality might have on criminal profiling proficiency. Although a variety of sources had at the time described criminal profiling as being applicable to crimes of arson *(20–22)*, no studies had previously examined the accuracy of criminal profiles for this type of crime. Indeed, consideration of this issue seemed particularly warranted in view of other studies *(23)*, which had found the applicability of some profiling principles to vary based on the considered crime modality. The second variation incorporated into this third study considered profiling proficiency within the specific context of recidivistic or serial crime. Although many authors have described profiling as most suited to crimes of a serial nature, in which patterns are likely to be manifested across the behaviors of a series of offenses *(22,24)*, all previous considerations of criminal profiling had involved single offense crimes.

The general design of this third study followed that of the two previous ones *(15,19)*. Thus, the first step in this study once again involved obtaining case materials. On this occasion, however, the materials originated from a police investigation into a large series of fires committed by an individual who could be viewed as a serial arsonist. Akin to the procedures used in the previous two studies, these case materials were summarized up to the point just before the offender's apprehension. Accompanying these materials was another multiple-choice questionnaire that was developed and allowed a participant to provide their predictions concerning the characteristics of the probable arsonist. Because this offense series had been solved, the identity of the arsonist was known, and a set of model answers for scoring the questionnaire was developed by using the answers of the chief detective involved in the case, who was intimately familiar with the offender's details. Akin to the two previous studies, these case materials and the questionnaire were then administered to various skill-based groups of participants and the accuracy of their predictions scored by the use of these model answers.

Although the first study *(15)* revealed some promising indications for the abilities of profilers, the findings were somewhat tentative. Additionally, those findings were in the context of profiling a murder. Because this third study considered a crime modality that had never been previously examined in a profiling experiment (i.e., serial arson), it was important to incorporate another sample of expert profilers to once again gauge their proficiency with regard to this particular crime modality.

In considering participants who would not only possess investigative experience, but also qualitatively relevant experience in the investigation of arson offenses, two separate groups of participants were obtained. The first group consisted of experienced police detectives who either worked exclusively in a specialist police arson investigation unit or who regularly investigated and had been trained to investigate arson offenses. Thus, it was hoped that this group would exemplify all dimensions of investigative experience by including detectives in the study who embodied both quantitative years of experience as well as qualitatively specific skills related to the investigation of arson crimes.

The second group gathered to test the importance of investigative experience were fire brigade arson investigators. These were not police officers but fire brigade officers who were specifically trained in the forensic chemical and physical examination of fire crime scenes to determine the possibility of whether a fire had been deliberately lit *(25)*. These participants typically worked in close conjunction with police detectives, but their investigative experiences focused more on the scientific examination of a fire scene to determine the probable cause and origin of a fire.

Consistent with the previous studies, a group of science students and a control group were also recruited. Given the surprising performance of the

Table 3.3
Mean Profile Accuracy Scores Between Groups

	Profilers ($n = 3$)	Police detectives ($n = 13$)	Arson investigators ($n = 12$)	Students ($n = 21$)	Controls (no case material; $n = 43$)
Total accuracy	$23^{a,b}$	16.23^{a}	17.67	19.52^{c}	$16.34^{b,c}$

^{a,b,c,d}Overall statistical differences are present between groups with specific pair-wise differences denoted by the same superscripted letter (e.g., *a* and *a*).

science student groups in the previous two studies it was important to again consider these participants who lacked investigative experience but who were instead adept at logical and objective analysis. Similarly, as a conceptual baseline of what could be achieved by relying on little more than guesswork and/or stereotypical conceptions, another control group was recruited who were only provided with the multiple-choice questionnaire and no case material. Once again, this control group was asked to answer the questionnaire by describing what they believed were the characteristics of the typical serial arsonist.

As previously mentioned, the questionnaire was administered to each of these groups. The completed questionnaires were collated for each of the respective groups, scored for accuracy, and then subjected to statistical analysis. The outcome of these analyses is summarized in Table 3.3 and in many respects the outcome is consistent with those of the previous two studies. First, looking at the descriptive patterns, the group that achieved the highest mean score in accurately predicting the characteristics of the serial arsonist were the profilers, thus providing another modicum of evidence for their superior capabilities. However, even more notable was that the profilers' degree of accuracy surpassed the police detectives to such an extent that it was found to be statistically significant. Consequently, this particular finding speaks favorably of the potential input of profilers to criminal investigations, because their predictions concerning a serial arsonist are likely to be significantly more accurate than what detectives themselves might predict.

Following the profilers, and generally consistent with the patterns of the previous study, the science students achieved the next highest accuracy score. Although not statistically distinct from the groups representative of investigative experience (i.e., police detectives and fire investigators), the mean score of the science students was nonetheless descriptively higher despite these participants not possessing any investigative experience whatsoever, and instead, having skills aligned with logical and objective reasoning. Finally, in considering the performance of the various groups in comparison with the control condition, only the profilers and science students were found to surpass the control group at a statistically significant level. Although surprising, this finding is consistent with those of the previous study in indicating that the detectives and arson investigators were unable to accurately predict the characteristics of the serial arsonist any better than what could have been achieved by simply guessing or relying on stereotypical conceptions.

In conclusion, the findings of this third study offer some promising, albeit modest, indications concerning the proficiency of expert profilers in predicting the characteristics of a serial arsonist. However, akin to its predecessor, the findings of this study lend little support to Hazelwood et al.'s *(14)* contentions concerning the importance, or even necessity, of investigative experience for an individual successfully engaging in the proficient construction of a criminal profile.

A Combined Analysis of All Studies

Although the findings of the three studies canvassed thus far *(15,19,26)* each offer some long overdue scrutiny of the accuracy of profilers, each featured comparatively modest samples. Additionally, these studies were undertaken independently and successively, and consequently, their findings are reflective of the respective data pools used for each study. It was considered a useful exercise therefore to combine the previously separate data sets from each of the three studies to gain a holistic impression of the performance of all groups in comparison with each other *(27)*. Additionally, such an analysis would also provide a good opportunity to include some previously unused data to assist in the statistical strength of this combined analysis.

Because the three studies considered different crimes and used different questionnaires (i.e., two studies on murder and one on arson), combining the data could not be accomplished by simply tallying together the values from each of the respective studies. Instead, a statistical procedure was needed to convert all data to an equivalent and comparable level. This process involved converting all scores into what are referred to as *z*-scores. Without delving into a statistical explanation of this process, the resulting values, as displayed in Table 3.4, can simply be interpreted by their proximity to the value of 1.00. The closer a value is to 1.00 the higher its accuracy. Conversely, values further away from 1.00 are indicative of a low level of accuracy.

The combination and analysis of these data sets as displayed in Table 3.4 represents the largest empirically based study that seeks to critically examine the comparative accuracy of different skill-based groups in construct-

*At the time of the publication of this book and to the best of the author's knowledge.

Table 3.4
Comparative Profile Accuracy Between Groups

	Profilers ($n = 11$)	Psychologists ($n = 36$)	Science students ($n = 85$)	Specialist detectives ($n = 25$)	General police ($n = 85$)	Police recruits ($n = 50$)	Non-police specialists ($n = 12$)	Psychics ($n = 20$)	Controls (no case material; $n = 120$)
Accuracy score	0.82	0.16	0.31	–0.43	0.07	0.17	0.12	–0.14	–0.36

Accuracy denoted by a value closest to 1.00. For example, 0.75 is indicative of a high level of accuracy, whereas –0.75 is indicative of low accuracy.

ing criminal profiles.* Consistent with the previous studies, the group that once again demonstrated the highest degree of accuracy was the expert profilers. Interestingly, however, and in contrast to the findings of the first study *(15)*, the next most proficient group were found to be the science students, followed by the psychologists. Among the various groups representative of differing levels of investigative experience the police recruits and the arson investigators performed the best, whereas other groups, such as the general duties police officers and specialist detectives, performed, comparatively speaking, quite poorly.

Conclusion

The studies discussed in this chapter should be viewed as a long overdue attempt to undertake a systematic and empirically based investigation of the skills and accuracy inherent to the proficient construction of criminal profiles. Although the findings of these studies provide some promising indications, they do not represent a definitive treatise on the topic. Further replication of these studies is clearly warranted involving larger groups of expert profilers and differing types of crimes as the subject of any profiling experiments. Nevertheless, the importance of these studies should not be underestimated. Although they may be perceived as simply reinforcing some commonly held views concerning the merits of criminal profiling, they nonetheless offer some long overdue empirical evidence in the form of a series of scientific experiments. Such experiments provide a systematic demonstration of criminal profiling that can be objectively and independently scrutinized and tested by others in the future.

In considering these studies, however, it is vital to appreciate their design parameters and their implications. In the field of criminal profiling, one notion that has acquired almost folklore status is the belief that predictions contained in criminal profiles, as constructed by personnel from a particular law enforcement organization, possess an approximately 80% degree of accuracy. The basis of this notion appears to originate from a personal communication cited in Pinizzotto *(28)* and seems to refer to research from an internal report that, at the time of publication and to the author's knowledge, is not available for independent public scrutiny *(29)*. What must be clearly recognized is that the experimental structure of the studies in this chapter *(15,19,20,27)* were not designed to measure, in quantifiable terms, the degree of accuracy in a criminal profile. That is, whether the responses on the questionnaires achieved, for example, a 50, 60, or even 80% degree of accuracy. These studies were designed solely for the purpose of conducting comparative analyses of the capabilities of various skill-based groups in accurately predicting, that is profiling, the characteristics of an unknown perpetrator(s) to a crime. Consequently, these studies should not in anyway be interpreted as relevant or indeed supportive of the notion of criminal profiles possessing an 80% degree of accuracy.

Instead, these studies should be viewed in terms of whether different skill-based groups are more adept at profiling than others. In this context, the present studies provide some support for the capabilities of expert profilers in accurately predicting the characteristics of an unknown offender following some assessment of the crime as compared with the other sampled groups. These findings, however, are not intended to provide any quantifiable indication of the margin by which profilers excel, nor do the studies attempt to indicate the degree of accuracy in percentage terms typically exhibited in the criminal profiles generated.

It is in this context of a comparative analysis that other important implications emerge from these studies regarding the skills most likely to be aligned to the proficient, (i.e., accurate) construction of a criminal profile. Possibly the clearest, and most likely controversial, implication is the lack of evidence to support the necessity of experience in law enforcement or more precisely, investigative experience for an individual to be able to accurately construct a criminal profile. This conclusion is derived from the consistently poor performance of the sampled police personnel in comparison with the other groups in these studies. Undoubtedly, this conclusion is one that is not likely to sit comfortably with some in the law enforcement community or indeed expert profilers who actively market their experience in law enforcement and/or investigations as their primary and most compelling asset *(30)*. For this reason it needs to be emphasized that the studies described throughout this chapter involved an objective and straightforward test. Various groups undertook this test and the outcomes of their performance were simply reported. Thus, the statistical analyses of these studies were not undertaken with any preconceived objectives or designs to favor one group over another.

Having indicated that these studies fail to support the need for investigative experience in constructing an accurate criminal profile, an important clarification is warranted. That is, this conclusion should not be misinterpreted as suggesting that criminal profiles cannot be constructed by law enforcement personnel. On the contrary, these studies merely indicate that there is no basis for there to be any need for prior experience in criminal investigations, or more broadly law enforcement, for an individual to be able to construct an accurate criminal profile.

Although individuals with varying degrees of investigative experience may engage in the construction of criminal profiles, these studies indicate that such experiences are unlikely to enhance their abilities in constructing an accurate profile.

In contrast to investigative experience, the skills most likely to be aligned with the accurate construction of a criminal profile appear to be sourced in an individual's understanding of human behavior (i.e., psychological skills), and more fundamentally, a capacity to examine and analyze material in a logical and objective manner. This is borne out by the consistently strong performance of the psychologists and more importantly, that of the science students in comparison with the other sampled groups. Consequently, it is the pursuit of these skills and/or knowledge base that should be paramount in selecting an individual to construct a criminal profile and, arguably, in selecting individuals to be trained in the construction of criminal profiles. Clearly, skills in understanding human behavior as well as logical and objective reasoning are not foreign to police personnel. Perhaps, however, police personnel who are engaged in constructing criminal profiles, or who wish to pursue training in the construction of criminal profiles, should be able to demonstrate these skills at an advanced level.

In conclusion, some measure of empirically robust evidence is now available to suggest that criminal profiles constructed by expert profilers are likely to possess a comparatively higher degree of accuracy in their predictions. Additionally, contrary to rhetoric, it appears the constituent skills most likely to be associated with the accurate construction of a criminal profile are not aligned necessarily with popular conceptions concerning the preeminence of investigative experience. Rather, the task of generating an accurate criminal profile is, in reality, more likely the product of one who has an appreciation of human behavior and is adept at logical, objective analysis.

References

1. Douglas, J.E. and Olshaker, M. (1995). Mindhunter. London: Heinman.
2. McCrary, G.O. and Ramsland, K. (2003). The unknown darkness: Profiling the predators among us. New York: Harper Collins.
3. Ressler, R.K. and Shachman, T. (1992). Whoever fights monsters. New York: Simon & Schuster.
4. Kocsis, R.N. and Palermo, G.B. (2005). Ten major problems with criminal profiling. Am J Forensic Psychiatry, 26(2), 45–67.
5. Kocsis, R.N. and Coleman, S. (2000). The unexplored ethics of criminal psychological profiling, In: Godwin, M.G., ed. Criminal psychology and forensic technology: A collaborative approach to effective profiling. New York: CRC Press, pp. 323–338.
6. Muller, D.A. (2000). Criminal profiling: Real science or just wishful thinking? Homicide Studies, 4(3), 234–264.

7. Copson, G. (1995). Coals to Newcastle: A study of offender profiling. London: Home Office.
8. Jackson, J.L., Van Koppen, P.J., Herbrink, C.M. (1993). Does the service meet the needs? An evaluation of consumer satisfaction with specific profile analysis and investigative advice offered by the scientific research advisory unit of the National Criminal Intelligence Division (CRI) (NISCALE Report NSCR 93-05). Amsterdam: NSCR.
9. Pinizzotto, A.J. (1984). Forensic psychology: Criminal personality profiling. Journal of Police Science and Administration, 12, 32–40.
10. Oleson, J.C. (1996). Psychological profiling: Does it actually work? Forensic Update, 46, 11–14.
11. Pinizzotto, A.J. and Finkel, N.J. (1990). Criminal personality profiling: An outcome and process study. Law of Human Behavior, 14, 215–233.
12. Douglas, J.E. and Burgess, A.W. (1986). Criminal profiling: A viable investigative tool against violent crime. FBI Law Enforcement Bulletin, 55(12), 9–13.
13. Ressler, R.K., Burgess, A., Douglas, J.E. (1988). Sexual homicide: Patterns and motives. New York: Lexington Books.
14. Hazelwood, R.R., Ressler, R.K., Depue, R.L., Douglas, J.C. (1995). Criminal investigative analysis: An overview. In: Hazelwood, R.R. and Burgess, A.W., eds. Practical aspects of rape investigation: A multidisciplinary approach, 2nd ed. Boca Raton, FL: CRC Press, pp. 115–126.
15. Kocsis, R.N., Irwin, H.J., Hayes, A.F., Nunn, R. (2000). Expertise in psychological profiling: A comparative assessment. Journal of Interpersonal Violence, 15(3), 311–331.
16. Harrower, J. (1998). Applying psychology to crime. London: Hodder & Stoughton.
17. Godwin, J. (1978). Murder USA: The ways we kill each other. New York: Ballantine.
18. Wilson, C. and Seaman, D. (1992). The serial killers. London: Cox & Wyman.
19. Kocsis, R.N., Hayes, A.F., Irwin, H.J. (2002). Investigative experience and accuracy in psychological profiling of a violent crime. Journal of Interpersonal Violence, 17(8), 811–823.
20. Holmes, R.M. and Holmes, S.T. (1996). Profiling violent crimes: An investigative tool, 2nd ed. Thousand Oaks, CA: Sage.
21. Rossmo, D.K. (1997). Geographic profiling. In: Jackson, J.L. and Bekerian, D., eds. Offender profiling: Theory, research and practice. London: Wiley, pp. 159–176.
22. Vorpagel, R.E. (1982). Painting psychological profiles: Charlatanism, coincidence, charisma or new science. Police Chief, 3(8), 156–159.
23. Kocsis, R.N. and Irwin, H.J. (1997). An analysis of spatial patterns in serial rape, arson, and burglary: The utility of the circle theory of environmental range for psychological profiling. Psychiatry, Psychology and Law, 4, 195–206.
24. Douglas, J.E., Ressler, R.K., Burgess, A.W., Hartman, C.R. (1986). Criminal profiling from crime scene analysis. Behavioral Science and Law, 4, 401–421.
25. DeHaan, J.D. (1991). Kirk's fire investigation, 3rd ed. Englewood Cliffs, NJ: Prentice Hall.
26. Kocsis, R.N. (2004). Psychological profiling of serial arson offenses: An assessment of skills and accuracy. Criminal Justice and Behavior, 31(3), 341–361.

27. Kocsis, R.N. (2003). Criminal psychological profiling: Validities and Abilities. International Journal of Offender Therapy and Comparative Criminology, 47(2), 126–144.
28. Pinizzotto, A.J. (1984). Forensic psychology: Criminal personality profiling. Journal of Police Science and Administration, 12(1), 32–40.
29. Institutional Research and Development Unit, FBI Academy. (1981). Evaluation of the psychological profiling program. Unpublished manuscript.
30. McCrary, G.O. (2003). Behavioral Criminology International website. Available from: http://www.criminalprofiler.com/index.htm. Accessed June 26, 2005.

Chapter 4

The Components and Processes of Criminal Profiling

Summary

Research in the area of criminal profiling has been largely preoccupied with the development of offender taxonomies and principles relevant to the profiling of violent crimes. Seemingly overlooked, however, has been any systematic and empirically based examination of the components and processes involved in the construction of a criminal profile. This chapter canvasses a series of studies that provide some tentative insights into these issues, including the information found within criminal profiles as constructed by expert profilers, the input of differing forms of case material, and the cognitive processes associated with the accurate construction of a criminal profile.

Key Words: Criminal profile content; construction processes; case materials.

Introduction

Chapter 3 addressed the paucity of empirically robust research surrounding the accuracy and constituent skills associated with criminal profiling. It highlighted that although some popular, albeit untested, notions exist, including the importance of investigative experience, the available empirical evidence may challenge such notions. In an analogous fashion, this chapter explores various issues surrounding the components and processes involved in the construction of criminal profiles that similarly attract populist notions but have largely escaped systematic empirical scrutiny to date.

In promoting the benefits of criminal profiles to police investigators, for example, a number of authors have identified differing types of information a profile may typically contain *(1,2)*. These include factors such as an offender's

From: *Criminal Profiling: Principles and Practice*
By: R. N. Kocsis © Humana Press Inc., Totowa, NJ

age, gender, race, marital status, or employment history. Surprisingly, however, little empirically based research has been undertaken that examines the kind of information actually contained in a criminal profile constructed by an expert profiler compared with one generated by another skill-based group.

Similarly, the processes involved in constructing a criminal profile have received remarkably little empirical investigation. Although it is commonly believed that criminal profiling involves intensive expert analysis of investigative case material, the literature in the field has failed to examine how differing forms of case material may affect this analysis and thus the construction of a criminal profile. For example, how much and what types of information are needed for the proficient (i.e., accurate) construction of a criminal profile? Additionally, systematic consideration of the cognitive functions involved in the assessment of case materials for the construction of a criminal profile has largely escaped study. For instance, what cognitive functions do expert profilers use that may account for their higher degree of proficiency in constructing a criminal profile? The studies summarized in this chapter were undertaken in an effort to answer some of these questions.

*The Content of Criminal Profiles**

One of the fundamental purposes of a criminal profile is to present information describing the characteristics of the probable offender of a crime. Various lists prescribing the types of information commonly thought to be contained in criminal profiles have been proposed *(1,2)*. However, very little literature exists that effectively examines the amount and type of information contained in a criminal profile constructed by an expert profiler as compared with any other author.

Possibly the only previous empirical study to consider these issues was undertaken by Pinizzotto and Finkel *(3)*. These researchers compared the content of profiles written by profilers with profiles written by small groups of police officers, psychologists, and university students. The results of their investigation were limited in that they simply indicated that profilers tended to write longer reports containing a larger number of predictions. It was this remarkable deficit of information that motivated the present study *(4)*, which sought to build on Pinizzotto and Finkel's *(3)* earlier findings by exploring the differences, if any, between the types of information contained in criminal profiles constructed by expert profilers and those constructed by others.

*It must once again be stated that for brevity and ease of comprehension, only abridged summaries of the various studies undertaken are canvassed in the context of this chapter.

This study *(4)* considered the survey form developed in the first study described in Chapter 3. In that previous study, a test instrument was devised that provided participants with a booklet summarizing the case material available to police immediately before the apprehension of the offender in a real murder case. As described in the previous chapter, this case information was accompanied by a questionnaire that was designed to elicit information from a respondent concerning their predictions (i.e., criminal profile) of the probable offender. The various studies in Chapter 3 focused on the data obtained from the responses to the multiple-choice questionnaires. However, one component of the first study discussed in Chapter 3 which was not previously analyzed, involved participants being given the opportunity to examine the case package and construct a written criminal profile.

Consequently, the present study examined the information contained in the written profiles generated by 5 expert profilers, 29 psychologists, 34 police officers, and 19 self-identified professional psychics (the groups of participants from the first study discussed in Chapter 3). This analysis was undertaken by first devising an extensive list of 39 items of information that could be articulated in a criminal profile.* This list of items was subdivided into three broad categories that included physical features (e.g., the offender's age, gender, or build), non-physical descriptive features (e.g., the offender's marital and religious status), and crime behaviors (e.g., whether the offender was previously familiar with the crime scene). Using this list, each of the criminal profiles composed by the profilers, police officers, university students, and psychics were carefully read and assigned a score for each of the 39 items they answered. In this way, their answers yielded a prediction in respect of each of the 39 items. As a methodological precaution to ensure the reliability of this scoring process, a second independent researcher separately re-read each profile and undertook the same scoring procedure, finally, the scores between the two researchers on each profile were cross checked. This procedure was necessary to safeguard the reliability of the obtained scores contained in each of the profiles.

After each of the criminal profiles had been scored according to the number of items they each contained, these scores were then tallied together for each of the respective groups and subjected to statistical analyses to determine if any differences existed in the information contained in the profiles. The results of this analysis are summarized in Table 4.1.

---

*Readers who wish to inspect this list may refer to the original manuscript by the author *(4)*.

Table 4.1
Number of Features Contained in Criminal Profiles Among Groups

	Profilers ($n = 5$)	Psychologists ($n = 29$)	Police ($n = 34$)	Students ($n = 27$)	Psychics ($n = 19$)
Total no. of words	Highest	Lower	Lower	Lower	Lower
Total no. of features	Highest	Lower	Lower	Lower	Lower
Physical features	Same (no sig. difference)	Same (no sig. difference)	Same (no sig. difference)	Same (no sig. difference)	Same (no sig. difference)
Nonphysical features	Highest	Lower	Lower	Lower	Lower
Features of crime	Highest/same (no sig. difference between profilers vs psychologists)	Highest/same (no sig. difference between profilers vs psychologists)	Lower	Lower	Lower

α/Significant differences at 0.05.

From a purely quantitative perspective, the results of this analysis indicate that the profiles written by the expert profilers contain more words* and predictions than the profiles written by any of the other groups. In effect, therefore, this finding accords with the observations made previously by Pinizzotto and Finkel *(3)*. What is perhaps more illuminating in terms of our understanding of criminal profiles, however, concerns the types of information found in the criminal profiles generated by each of the different groups. The profiles constructed by the expert profilers generally contained more information relating to the crime behaviors and non-physical descriptive features of the probable offender than any† of the compared groups. However, no statistically significant differences were found in the amount of information concerning the offender's physical features that the expert profilers predicted in comparison with any of the other groups. Consequently, the findings of this study highlight that beyond simply being larger with more predictions, criminal profiles written by expert profilers tend to specifically contain more information relating to crime behaviors and the background history of the likely offender.

Case Materials and Criminal Profile Construction

The previous study offered some insight into the amount and types of information expert profilers provide within the context of a written criminal profile. However, the study did not investigate how these criminal profiles were constructed. More specifically, what mechanisms, processes, or cognitive functions are involved with the proficient (i.e., accurate) construction of a profile? The next two studies sought to investigate these issues.

It seems reasonable to assume that a relationship probably exists between the type of case materials available and the way such materials are assessed for the purpose of constructing a criminal profile. For example, in the study by Pinizzotto and Finkel *(3)*, differences in the case materials for the rape and murder offenses (the subject of their respective profiling experiments) were suggested as possibly accounting for the poor performance of the profilers in the murder profiling exercise. Indeed, expert profilers are frequently noted to place considerable emphasis on the availability of case materials for the profi-

*This particular aspect of each profile involved the verbatim retyping of each word contained in the criminal profile into a computer word processor and then using the word count function.

†One exception being the expert profilers and the psychologists. Although the profilers descriptively surpassed the psychologists in the crime behaviors measure, this difference was not found to be statistically significant.

cient construction of a criminal profile. In articulating a procedural model by which criminal profiles may be constructed, Douglas et al. *(5)*, for example, emphasize the importance of case materials and their cyclic re-evaluation for the construction of a criminal profile.

Consequently, as a starting point for exploring the mechanisms involved in the construction of a criminal profile, examination of the influence, if any, case materials may have on the accurate construction of a profile was considered. It was this issue the second study set out to investigate *(6)*. Given the nature of this study, it was assumed that most material compiled during a criminal investigation could be categorized into one of two types of information: visual or narrative case materials.* Visual material in the context of the study refers to graphical material that generally depicts physical aspects of a human being, object, or place and thus includes, but is not limited to, such things as schematic diagrams and photographs of any autopsy or crime scene *(6)*. In a similar vein, narrative material is defined as any information communicated in some type of written format and thus includes, but is again not limited to, such items as police, forensic expert, or witness statements.

A simple test of the influence these differing forms of case material might have involves the segregation of case materials by this distinction and observing any differences this segregation may have on the proficient (i.e., accurate) construction of a criminal profile. This would involve using the survey form described in the first study in Chapter 3. As previously explained, this survey instrument contained a case package summarizing the case materials compiled by an actual police investigation into a murder. Adjoining this case package was a 33-item multiple-choice questionnaire whereby a participant could provide their profile of the probable perpetrator of a murder that was the subject of the case file materials. The accuracy of their responses in predicting the unknown murderer's characteristics were then objectively scored via the use of a set of model answers to the questionnaire describing the offender's characteristics.

Thus, this same survey instrument was again used, however, the case materials that previously preceded the multiple-choice questionnaire were separated and were either present or absent among the material supplied to participants depending on whether they were of a visual or narrative nature. Consequently, this second study created four versions of the survey form, each

*It is acknowledged that this represents a simplistic distinction and that other forms of case material may be generated during the course of a police investigation that would not comfortably sit with this dichotomy. Nonetheless, for the purpose of this initial study, given the material typically compiled and assessed by profilers *(2)*, this distinction was adopted.

dependent on the type of case material they contained. The first version was the "full" questionnaire, effectively representing the survey form as administered in the first study discussed in Chapter 3 wherein all case materials just before the apprehension of the actual murderer were provided to the participant. Accordingly, this version of the survey form demonstrated what could be achieved with the presence of all case materials. The second version of the survey instrument was the "narrative only" condition and in this case all visual materials were removed from the survey instrument. Thus, this version of the survey form contained only written case material. This version therefore served as a demonstration of what could be achieved in terms of profiling the offender with only the written materials available. The reverse of this was the "visual only" condition. As denoted by its title, this version only contained visual case materials and consequently served as a demonstration of what could be achieved through the use of the visual case materials only. Finally, to act as a hybrid between the visual and narrative only conditions, another condition was created that contained the narrative case material with written descriptions of the features depicted in each item of the visual material.

Consequently, the study's participants completed one of the four versions of the survey instrument. The differences in terms of profile accuracy in completing these different versions of the survey form could then be traced to the differences in the source material. As a final nuance, a fifth control condition was also incorporated that was akin to the control conditions used in the studies described in Chapter 3. This control condition simply presented participants with the multiple-choice questionnaire minus any case material to provide an indication of what could be accomplished in terms of responding to the questionnaire by merely guessing and/or relying on stereotypical conceptions of a typical murderer.

Because the factor being tested in this study was the influence of the case materials, it was important to keep, where possible, all other factors constant. The studies in Chapter 3 used differing skill-based groups of participants to observe the contributions of those identified skills for the accurate construction of a criminal profile. However, because the differences in the case materials supplied were the examined variable in this study, it was important that all participants possessed a relatively equal skill basis. Compounding this concern was the logistical aspect of obtaining a sufficient number of people to participate in this study. Because the number of expert profilers is relatively small, another homogeneously skilled group was needed. Based on their logistical availability and their ability to profile crimes (as denoted by the studies canvassed in Chapter 3), a sample of 122 science sophomores was recruited. In summary, therefore, this study involved one of five different versions of the survey form being randomly admistered to each of these students. Analogous to all of the previous studies in Chapter 3, the responses on each of the questionnaires were scored for accuracy and then tallied together for their respective versions and subjected to statistical analyses to identify any differences. The results of this analysis are summarized in Table 4.2.

Two important findings emerge from this analysis. First, the results demonstrate the importance of having all case materials available for the accurate construction of a criminal profile. From a purely descriptive perspective, all of the groups who were provided with at least some case materials surpassed the control group, which merely guessed and/or relied on stereotypical notions of a murderer in responding to the questionnaire. However, the only group that surpassed the control condition at a statistically significant level was the group that was provided with all case materials. Consequently, this finding indicates, perhaps unsurprisingly, that the proficient construction of a criminal profile is clearly related to the availability of more, rather than less, case material. Indeed, the optimal circumstance for the construction of a criminal profile (measured purely in terms of accuracy) is likely to be achieved when all forms of case materials are present.

The second and more subtle finding to emerge relates to the impact that differing types of case material are likely to have on the accurate construction of a criminal profile. Specifically, the score of the group, which was provided with only narrative case materials, was higher than that of the group provided with only visual materials. Indeed, the score of the narrative only condition is close to that of the group who possessed all case materials. Consequently, there is some evidence to suggest that case material in the narrative form has a greater role in the process of constructing an accurate criminal profile.

Cognitive Processes in Constructing a Criminal Profile

Whereas the first study *(4)* provided some impression of the information contained in criminal profiles as composed by expert profilers and the second study *(6)* examined the influence of case materials, neither considered the cognitive processes likely to be associated with the construction of a criminal profile. Specifically, what mental functions may account for the comparatively higher degree of accuracy expert profilers appear to demonstrate in predicting the characteristics of an unknown offender?

Although not representative of these cognitive functions, a number of authors *(5,7–9)* have proposed various procedural models for how a criminal profile should be composed via the analysis of case information. It appears these models largely lack empirical basis and are more informed by the vari-

Table 4.2
Mean Profile Accuracy Scores as Measured by Varying Amounts of Case Material

	All case material ($n = 22$)	Narrative only ($n = 20$)	Narrative with descriptions ($n = 20$)	Visual only ($n = 20$)	Control (no case material) ($n = 40$)	p-value
Accuracy scores	12.22[a]	11.95	10.25	10.75	10.20[a]	0.05 (sig. differences)

[a]Pair-wise significant differences.
α-levels at 0.05.

ous authors' anecdotal experiences and/or observations. Unsurprisingly, therefore, little consistency exists among these models with one exception. All models appear to assume that the mental assimilation of case information, presumably via memory, is an integral component of the mental processes involved in the accurate construction of a criminal profile.

Possibly the only previous study to undertake some empirical investigation of the cognitive processes associated with the construction of a criminal profile was that by Pinizzotto and Finkel *(3)*. These authors also viewed the cognitive assimilation of case material as integral to profile construction. As previously discussed, Pinizzotto and Finkel's *(3)* research compared small skill-based groups of participants in various profiling exercises involving a murder and rape case. In completing these exercises, a participant's recollection of the facts of the case was also tested. A number of interesting, although perplexing, findings emerged from their experiments. Although the sampled profilers did not exhibit any superiority in accurately predicting the characteristics of the unknown murderer, they nonetheless recalled a significantly greater amount of information about the murder case. Ironically, although the profilers demonstrated some superiority in predicting the characteristics of the rapist, they did not display any superiority in the amount of information they could recall from the rape case. In discussing their findings, Pinizzotto and Finkel *(3)* concluded that one of the most distinguishing features related to the cognitive functions of profilers was not their capacity to recall details of any particular case, but rather, their ability to identify information that they regarded as relevant for constructing a profile.

Consequently, a third study was undertaken that sought to build on Pinizzotto and Finkel's earlier findings by examining a variety of the cognitive functions that were likely to underpin the construction of a criminal profile. To undertake such an experiment the test instruments used in both the murder and arson profiling studies discussed in Chapter 3 were again used. Aside from testing a respondent's ability to complete these forms, some additional tasks were developed to allow for some measurement of the cognitive functions associated with formulating predictions using the two types of survey forms.

Therefore, in addition to both the original murder and arson survey forms, a separate questionnaire was also included, which the respondent was required to answer immediately after they had completed the initial questionnaire. One important difference was that the various sections of the questionnaires were to be completed and sealed in an envelope before a participant could progress to answer the next section. Consequently, participants were instructed to complete these additional sections of the experiment without the benefit of referring back to the case materials or their previous profile.

The additional sections of the survey form primarily involved a participant completing three separate tasks. The first task asked respondents to simply write down as many items of information they could remember concerning the case they had just examined. Once they had completed this, the second task then required the respondents review this list of items and identify as many that they considered as important to the construction of a criminal profile as they could. The third and final task then presented the respondents with 40 questions concerning the case. These questions were not related to the identity of the probable offender but were focused on ascertaining respondents' comprehension of the case material they had just examined. The correct answers to all of these questions were evident in the previously examined case material that was now sealed in an envelope. Consequently, the scoring of these questions was accomplished by simply developing a set of model answers by referring to the case materials from which the questions were derived. Similarly, the scoring of the initial test in recalling as many items of information was achieved by simply tallying up the number of items a respondent noted and then verifying that each of them were indeed present by referring to the case materials.

This third study therefore involved two survey forms: one with respect to the murder case and the other with respect to the arson case as previously described in Chapter 3. Attached to each of the survey forms were now two additional questionnaires that gauged a participant's recollection and comprehension of the case material they had originally examined. By this procedure, some comparison could be made between a respondent's capabilities in profiling the characteristics of the unknown offender and their appreciation of the case information they had examined.

Two small groups of participants were obtained for this study, consisting of five expert profilers and five non-profilers (i.e., another sample of science students) to highlight the differences, if any, in their capacity to profile the unknown offender(s) and the role that memory and comprehension plays in such a profiling task. All members of the two groups completed both versions of the survey form. Their responses to the survey forms were scored, tallied, and subjected to statistical analysis as previously detailed. The results of these analyses are summarized in Tables 4.3 and 4.4.

Although not displayed in Tables 4.3 or 4.4, the first component of this analysis examined the proficiency of the expert profilers and non-profilers in accurately predicting the characteristics of the unknown offenders. Consistent with the findings discussed in Chapter 3, the profilers surpassed the non-profilers in correctly predicting the characteristics of the unknown offenders.*

---

*Readers interested in a more comprehensive analysis are recommended to refer to the original manuscript by Kocsis, Middledorp, and Try *(10)*.

Table 4.3
Summary of Relationship Between Profile Accuracy and Amounts of Recalled Case Information, Items Nominated as Relevant for Profile Composition, and Comprehension Questions Answered Correctly

	Recalled information		Nominated items		Comprehension questions	
	Murder	Arson	Murder	Arson	Murder	Arson
Profile accuracy	No relationship	No relationship	No relationship	Incremental relationship	Incremental relationship	Incremental relationship

Table 4.4
Comparison of Mean Comprehension Scores Between Profilers and Non-Profilers on Murder and Arson Cases

		Profilers	Non-profilers	*p*-Values
Comprehension questions (answered correctly)	Murder	32.8	28.8	0.071[a]
	Arson	33.4	23.6	0.001[a]

[a]Denotes statistically significant difference at α level of 0.10.

Although this offers another modicum of empirical evidence in support of the comparative proficiency of expert profilers, this result more importantly serves as a benchmark for investigating the cognitive functions associated with proficient profiling. That is, recognizing that expert profilers achieve a comparatively higher degree of accuracy in their predictions, what is it that they do differently, in comparison with the non-profilers, in terms of their cognitive functions?

Some indication of an answer to this question appears in Table 4.3, which summarizes the general relationship between profile accuracy and the amount of recalled case information, case information nominated as relevant, and the number of correctly answered questions. As indicated in Table 4.3, no relationship was found on either the murder or arson cases between the amount of case information the participants could recollect and the accuracy of their criminal profiles. Accordingly, it would appear that one cognitive function that does not appear to be related to proficient (i.e., accurate) profiling is the mere amount of case information an individual can recollect. Somewhat mixed findings, however, emerge with respect to profiling accuracy and the number of items nominated as relevant to profile construction. In this circumstance, a statistically significant incremental relationship was found to exist but only in the context of the arson case. Consequently, this finding offers some support for the earlier observation of Pinizzotto and Finkel *(3)*, which noted that profiler abilities seem to be related to their capacity to identify certain items of case information.

The most prominent result to emerge, however, concerned the patterns between profiling accuracy and the comprehension of the case materials as measured by the respective score each participant achieved in correctly answering the 40 questions designed to measure comprehension of the case material. In this regard, a statistically significant incremental relationship was found to exist between accuracy and comprehension in both the murder and arson cases. That is, the higher the level of comprehension of the case material, the more accurate a profile was found to be. This finding provides some evidence to suggest that at least one cognitive function closely aligned to the accurate construction of a criminal profile is an individual's ability to comprehend the case material.

When considering the question of what might explain the comparatively superior degree of accuracy found among the expert profilers, the results summarized in Table 4.4 should be consulted. Although Table 4.3 indicates the existence of a general conceptual relationship between profiling accuracy and comprehension, Table 4.4 suggests that it is indeed this particular cognitive function that accounts for the superior accuracy of profilers. In this context, Table 4.4 compares the mean scores of the comprehension questionnaire of the expert profilers with the non-profilers in the murder and arson cases. In both circumstances the expert profilers consistently achieved higher comprehension scores and this superiority was found to be statistically significant at varying levels. Consequently, at least one cognitive function amongst the sampled profilers that may account for their superior ability to accurately profile the characteristics of an unknown offender may indeed be their capacity to better comprehend case material.

Conclusion

What should be apparent from these studies is that the construction of a criminal profile appears to be influenced by a host of contextual factors of which only a few have been examined by the studies briefly canvassed in this chapter. This is important to appreciate because in many respects the components and mechanisms associated with the construction of an accurate criminal profile are analogous to the construction of a sound psychiatric or psychological report, which typically involves interview, analysis, diagnosis, and the generation of a report *(11)*. Unlike the disciplines of psychiatry or psychology, however, which pay considerable attention to developing conventions and criteria for accepted practice among practitioners *(12–14)*, the field of criminal profiling seems devoid of such guiding principles especially regarding the practical construction of a robust criminal profile.

Accordingly, the significance of these preliminary studies should not be underestimated. The fact that a criminal profile, as constructed by an expert profiler, is likely to be larger than that generated by an individual from another skill-based group does not seem particularly enlightening. Indeed, quantity does not necessarily equate with quality in terms of the accuracy of a criminal profile. The ideal criminal profile should arguably be succinct and insightful in identifying potential suspects. Nonetheless, when considered alongside the findings discussed in Chapter 3, some relationship appears to exist between quantity and accuracy among the sampled profilers.

Importantly, however, the greatest contribution that a profile constructed by an expert profiler is likely to make is not in the provision of information concerning an offender's physical characteristics, but rather, information concerning psychological factors surrounding the crime and more specifically its perpetrator(s). This finding appears to accord with various studies that demonstrate surveyed police officers' satisfaction with criminal profiles. The findings of these surveys have often indicated that although profiles are not unreservedly endorsed as assisting in the identification of the offender, they are nonetheless often appreciated by investigators for the greater insight they offer into a crime, such as the offender's background history *(15,16)*.

Possibly the best demonstration of the impact of contextual factors on the accurate construction of a criminal profile can be discerned from the influence certain case materials appear to yield. Although it seems that optimal profiling is likely to be achieved when all forms of case material are available and this appears both logical and somewhat unsurprising, there is some suggestion that case material manifested in a narrative form plays a greater role in constructing an accurate criminal profile. Although this is only a tentative observation, it nonetheless has some interesting implications for both the practical construction of profiles and the cognitive processes involved with profiling. This appears to be at odds with popular fictional depictions of how expert profilers construct a profile. In fictional accounts, profilers are frequently portrayed as routinely requiring visits to crimes scenes and personal interviews of witnesses. Although the author does not argue against the potential benefits of such first-hand knowledge, such measures are often logistically impractical. The findings of the present study, however, offer some encouraging indications that the construction of an accurate profile may be largely dependent on the amount of narrative information available concerning the crime.

Aligned to these issues are the findings concerning the cognitive processes associated with criminal profiling. It seems that an incremental relationship exists between profiling accuracy and the comprehension of case material. Indeed, the data thus far suggests that it is this particular cognitive function of comprehension that expert profilers appear to excel in and that may in turn account, in part, for their comparatively superior ability in profiling the characteristics of an unknown offender(s) in the studies discussed thus far.

In conclusion, the studies in this chapter have examined only a few of the contextual factors surrounding the accuracy and construction of criminal profiles. These preliminary investigations offer some insight into what has been largely unexplored in profiling and highlights the need for greater scientific inquiry in this area. Clearly, more consideration of these issues in the form of carefully controlled and empirically driven studies is warranted.

References

1. Holmes, R.M. and Holmes, S.T. (1996). Profiling violent crimes: An investigative tool, 2nd ed. Thousand Oaks, CA: Sage.
2. Vorpagel, R.E. (1982). Painting psychological profiles: Charlatanism, coincidence, charisma or new science. Police Chief, 3(8), 156–159.
3. Pinizzotto, A.J. and Finkel, N.J. (1990). Criminal personality profiling: An outcome and process study. Law and Human Behavior, 14, 215–233.
4. Kocsis, R.N. (2003). An empirical assessment of content in criminal psychological profiles. International Journal of Offender Therapy and Comparative Criminology, 47(1), 38–47.
5. Douglas, J.E., Ressler, R.K., Burgess, A.W., Hartman, C.R. (1986). Criminal profiling from crime scene analysis. Behavioral Science and the Law, 4, 401–421.
6. Kocsis, R.N., Heller, G.Z., Try, A. (2003). Visual vs. narrative case material: Their impact on criminal psychological profiling? International Journal of Offender Therapy and Comparative Criminology, 47(4), 8–27.
7. Rossi, D. (1982). Crime scene behavioral analysis: Another tool for the law enforcement investigator. Police Chief, 18(4), 152–155.
8. Dietz, P.E. (1985). Sex offender profiling by the FBI: A preliminary conceptual model. In: Ben-Aron, M.H., Hucher, S.J., Webster, C.D., eds. Clinical criminology. Toronto: M & M Graphics, pp. 207–219.
9. Copson, G., Badcock, R., Boon, J., Britton, P. (1997). Articulating a systematic approach to clinical crime profiling. Criminal Behavior and Mental Health, 7, 13–17.
10. Kocsis, R.N., Middledorp, J., Try, A. (2005). Cognitive processes in criminal profile construction: A preliminary study. International Journal of Offender Therapy and Comparative Criminology, 49(6), 662–681.
11. Palermo, G.B. and Kocsis, R.N. (2005). Offender profiling: An introduction to the sociopsychological analysis of violent crime. IL: CC Thomas.
12. Shea, S.C. (1998). Psychiatric interviewing: The art of understanding. A practical guide for psychiatrists, psychologists, counselors, social workers, nurses and other mental health professionals, 2nd ed. Philadelphia: W.B. Saunders Company.
13. Morrison, J. (1995). DSM-IV made easy: The clinician's guide to diagnosis. New York: Guilford Press.
14. Zuckerman, E.L. (1995). Clinician's thesaurus: The guidebook for writing psychological reports, 4th ed. New York: Guilford Press.
15. Jackson, J.L, Van Hoppen, P.J., Hebrink, J. (1993). Does the service meet the needs? Amsterdam: Netherlands Institute for the Study of Criminality.
16. Pinizzotto, A.J. (1984). Forensic psychology: Criminal personality profiling. Journal of Police Science and Administration, 12(1), 32–40.

Chapter 5

Defining Serial Violent Crime

Summary

A redefinition of the term *serial crime* is pursued in this chapter by first identifying the psychological mechanisms characteristic of serial offenders; in this context, specific attention is given to the personality characteristics of psychopathy, narcissism, sadism, paraphilic tendencies, fantasy proneness or dissociative tendencies, and compulsiveness. A general definition of serial crime is proposed, focusing on the psychology of the serial offender regardless of the particular offense mode. As a result of this analysis, serial murder, serial rape, and serial arson can be described in terms of specific behaviors evidenced in the crime scene and the style of victimization; these descriptions may be used to classify serial offenders. It is this definition of serial crime that the Crime Action Profiling (CAP) studies adopt and, it is maintained, are likely to be indicative of the types of offenses that will practically benefit from the use of criminal profiling in their investigation.

Key Words: Definitions; serial violent crimes; sexual murder; serial arson; rape.

Introduction

In to order discuss the criminal profiling of serial violent crimes in any coherent manner, it is first necessary to understand what exactly is meant by the term *serial violent crime*. Although a seemingly elementary issue of terminology, the use of this term has implications for the methodological parameters followed in the sample collection of differing studies as well as for highlighting an important ideological difference in the Crime Action Profiling (CAP) research.

Accompanying the popularity of criminal profiling has been profiling research examining crimes that, in the pragmatic context of operational policing, often do not warrant the use of profiling. For example, a study by Salfati *(1)* examines the behavioral patterns and offender characteristics inherent to

From: *Criminal Profiling: Principles and Practice*
By: R. N. Kocsis © Humana Press Inc., Totowa, NJ

domestic homicides. Although this study represents a commendable contribution to the body of academic literature on the topic of domestic homicide, the utility of this study in the context of profiling is debatable because such offenses are often resolved through conventional investigative methods *(2,3)*. It appears that researchers are increasingly focusing on data that is readily accessible, at the expense of examining data that although not as accessible, is more relevant to the operational use and application of criminal profiles. That is, criminal profiling specifically evolved as a tool to assist in the investigation of crimes that were not readily resolvable through conventional investigative techniques *(4,5)*. Consequently, the generation of profiling research on crimes that generally do not necessitate profiling for their resolution in most circumstances seems something of a redundant exercise. One distinguishing ideological feature of the CAP research is that it specifically focuses on crimes that are not typically amenable to conventional investigative methods (such as those of a serial/sexual violent nature) that practically benefit from the use of criminal profiles. Consequently, it is important to carefully consider what, in terms of the CAP research, constitutes serial crime.

Unfortunately, coherence is lacking in the scholarly literature on defining serial crime. In the writings on serial murder, for example, there are differences of opinion as to whether serial murder represents an integral offense classification or a generic expression encompassing a variety of different offenses. In the *Crime Classification Manual (6)*, serial murder is designated as a discrete category of sexual homicide. However, researchers such as Holmes and Holmes *(7)* posit four different types of serial murderer, while Hickey *(8)* has proposed up to eight distinct categories.

It might be argued that differing typologies of serial murder do not necessarily detract from the coherence of an underlying concept. That is, notwithstanding various possible types of serial murder, some common factor(s) of this class of crime exist that render it immediately understood. The nature of any such common understanding, and in particular, the differentiation of serial murder from closely related crimes, nevertheless warrants closer scrutiny particularly when seeking to define serial violent crime.

Victim Numbers and Serial Crime

One may think a common feature of the term serial crime relates to the number of victims involved. Indeed, it is fair to say that the criterion of a minimum tally of victims has been the subject of debate in the conceptualization of serial crime. Rather surprisingly, however, there is much diversity in the empirical literature on serial crime regarding the minimum victim tally needed.

The number of victims used as the criterion for the classification of serial offenses has varied across agencies and researchers. For example, the North America National Institute of Justice defines serial murder as involving "two or more victims" *(9)*. In relation to serial rape, however, the procedural criterion applied in selecting cases for Canter and Larkin's *(10)* research project was a minimum of two victims of the same rapist. Others regard two offenses as not being sufficient to signify seriality. The FBI classifies serial crime (be it murder, rape, or arson) as at least three such offenses by the same person or persons *(6,11)*, whereas Hickey *(12)* has suggested that serial murder should be defined by a minimum of four victims. The rationale for any quantitative criteria is usually not explicit, although in the case of the FBI the criterion is presumably based on investigative experience. In any event, the lack of consistency in this regard impedes comparison and integration of the findings of different researchers. More fundamentally, however, there are substantial conceptual and practical difficulties in seeking to define serial crime purely in terms of a specific tally of victims or offenses.

A definition of serial crime solely in terms of offense numbers is insufficient to differentiate such crime from other types of crime entailing multiple offenses. Before 1980, there was no specific term for serial murders or serial crimes in general. Serial murders, for example, were simply grouped with any murder that involved several victims and referred to as mass murder. More recently, multiple murders have been differentiated into three categories: mass, spree, and serial murders *(5)*. The killing of three or more victims in a single event is now termed *mass murder (8,13–16)*, and the killing of three or more victims in different locations but within the context of the one event is referred to as *spree murder (5,6)*. According to FBI researchers *(6,11)*, *serial murder* is distinguished from these other forms of multiple murder in that it entails the murder of three or more victims with an intermission between each murder. Therefore, a definition of serial crime in terms of offense numbers would require at least supplementation by a temporal criterion to distinguish it from other crimes also characterized by multiple victims.

On the other hand, even when there is an intermission between multiple offenses, there are some crimes that are not usually regarded as serial. The so-called contract killer, for example, may murder several people in a similar manner over a period of time with an intermission and yet most criminologists would not regard this offender as a serial murderer *(17)*. Similarly, a hired torch may be responsible for several incidents of arson but would not usually be deemed a serial arsonist. The rationale for these distinctions is discussed in more detail later, but a definition of seriality simply in terms of a minimum number of offenses could be both over- and underinclusive.

A practical limitation of using minimum offense numbers is that for any given offender, the number of offenses known by authorities may be less than the number of offenses actually committed by that person. Police investigations often reveal additional offenses that are believed to have been committed by an arrested person but for which the evidence is insufficient to sustain a conviction *(18,19)*. Also, incarcerated offenders frequently boast of unaccounted for victims that have either eluded detection or identification by law enforcement agencies. For example, American serial killer Ted Bundy traded information about his undetected murders for delays in his execution *(20)*. Given that there are good reasons for believing that some serial criminals have committed more offenses than those for which they are charged, it would be inappropriate to assume that a person found guilty of only a single offense could not be a serial offender. In this respect, the definition of serial crime in terms of known offense numbers could be said to be potentially underinclusive.

There are other reasons, however, for rejecting a wholly number-based definition of serial sexual crime, if one considers the origins of the term. The term *serial* is derived from the word series and thus pertains to *"a group or connected succession of similar or related things usually arranged in order"* (*21*, p. 1412). It was in this sense of describing a succession of similar murders by the same offender(s) that the former FBI agent Robert Ressler popularized the expression serial killer *(22)*. In an attempt to operationalize this concept, it seems researchers have become distracted by the exercise of identifying a minimum offense tally to define serial crimes. This debate has served only to obscure the original meaning, namely, that the underlying characteristic of the serial offender is a psychological propensity to re-offend in a similar pattern. It is simply as an observed consequence of these persistent psychodynamics that this type of offender tends to accumulate multiple victims. Therefore, it is not the mere *post hoc* tally of offenses but the basis of the propensity to re-offend, a distinctive internal drive mechanism, that is quintessential to understanding and defining serial crime especially regarding serial sexual crime, which, it is argued, is most amenable to criminal profiling.

The propensity approach to serial violent crime illuminates the ways in which the term *serial* is applied. It is clear, for example, that in referring to serial crime, writers are not merely seeking to signify the presence of multiple offenses; rather, there is often an additional if implicit assumption about the psychological mechanisms of the offender. Thus, the term *serial* is not generally applied to just any sequence of similar offenses by the same person(s). A person who commits numerous thefts might commonly be described as a habitual thief but is generally not referred to as a serial thief. Indeed, the only crimes that commentators seem consistently to label as serial involve particular types of multiple offenses of murder, rape, or arson. Evidently, there is a specific inner drive assumed to be operating in these contexts, one that is thought, for example, not to be applicable to a sequential number of thefts. Thus, it is the basis of the psychological propensity to re-offend that seems to comprise the common understanding associated with the use of the expression "serial" with regard to crime. If serial crime is distinctive by its underlying psychodynamics, it is more properly defined in these terms than by a minimum offense tally.

The conceptualization of serial crime in terms of specific psychological propensities also clarifies distinctions often drawn between a series of crimes and similar cases in which there are multiple victims or targets. Thus, the contract killer and the hired torch are not regarded as serial criminals because their propensity to re-offend apparently is rooted in criminal enterprise or profit, and this motive does not accord with the implicit psychological drive of a serial criminal. In a similar fashion, consider the matter of multiple murder. It has been proposed that serial murder can be distinguished from mass murder and spree murder in terms of the factor of time or intermittence *(6,11)*. But there is also an assumption of a different psychology operating in each of these types of multiple murder. This is not to say there are no psychological similarities among the three types. It is often argued, for example, that all are senseless in that material gain is not involved, and that none resemble the broad patterns of murder generally observed *(2,3)*. Despite these similarities, however, the differentiation of serial murder from other types of mass murder is widely taken to imply the operation of a unique psychological etiology. That is, mass, spree, and serial murderers are thought to be driven by different psychodynamics. Whereas mass and spree murderers are deemed to be driven by life pressures, rage, and personality problems to a cathartic act of retribution, serial murder is often conceived as a remorseless pursuit of sexually based gratification, an on-going perverse and sadistic hobby *(6,11)*. Therefore, the psychological basis of a propensity to re-offend is more telling than any victim tally or time continuity in differentiating serial crime from similar offenses with multiple victims.

If crimes of serial homicide, rape, and arson are defined in terms of psychological propensities, however, there is a possibility that the term serial in this context is strictly a misnomer. That is, if evidence of the defining propensity is available, it might well be possible to classify an offender as serial without any evidence whatsoever that more than one offense has been committed by that person. Some instances in which this could be the case are considered here.

Serial Criminals Without Serial Offenses

The number of victims accrued by an offender will depend in part on factors other than the propensity to re-offend. An offender might possess the intrinsic psychological attributes of a serial offender, but could be prevented from offending more than once by, for example, illness or early apprehension by police. Indeed, Jenkins *(23)* has hypothesized that the accrual of victims is more a factor of the police response to the offenses than that of the offender's activities. In a hypothetical example, the victim tally might be relatively small if a serial murderer chose police officers as targets. Given the difficulties of getting the better of a police officer in an aggressive confrontation, as well as the probable vigor of the police response to the murder of one of their own, it seems improbable that such an offender would survive long enough to accumulate more than one victim. On the other hand, a killer who targeted prostitutes would perhaps be more likely to accrue numerous victims before being apprehended. There are circumstances, therefore, that may limit a criminal to a single offense, yet that person could still have the psychological characteristics of seriality; a particular type of propensity to re-offend.

By way of illustration, in Australia there have been several instances of a single murder case in which the style of victimization would be considered characteristic of a serial sexual murderer *(24)*. Barrie Watts and Valmae Beck, for example, exhibited the intrinsic features of serial murderers, yet Sian Kingi was their only victim before they were apprehended. In police statements, Watts openly expressed his earnest intentions to commit further murders. Furthermore, both Beck and Watts were apprehended while trawling for their next victim *(25)*. If there is some evidence of potential to re-offend it may therefore be possible to identify a serial criminal before more than one offense is committed. By focusing on the basis of the propensity to re-offend rather than on actual victim numbers, we also avoid the absurdity of implying that a serial killer is an intrinsically different sort of offender only after the commission of multiple offenses.

To the extent that a criminal may be categorized as serial when only one offense has been committed renders the expression serial crime a misnomer. In light of the wide usage of the expression, it seems almost futile to propose alternative, more appropriate terminology. The most viable solution may be the development of a satisfactory definition of serial crime. In this regard it is argued that the quintessential quality of serial crime lies in a particular type of propensity to re-offend. As discussed, a disposition to re-offend might well be evidenced by subsequent offenses, but it might also be evidenced by an offender's declaration of intent or by the offender's style of victimization (even in the initial offense[s]). The last of these possibilities requires exploration of the psychodynamics of a serial criminal, and in turn, the formulation of an effective definition of serial crime.

Psychological Factors in Serial Crime

A substantial portion of the empirical research concerning the psychological factors inherent in serial crime has focused on serial murder. The same emphasis on serial murder is placed in the present discussion, although some accounts of serial rape and serial arson are also given. By identifying the peculiar psychological mechanisms inherent in serial murder, not only can this offense be better understood, but also more generic manifestations of serial crime irrespective of whether that crime is murder, rape, or arson.

Psychological factors inherent to serial crime should not be taken to imply the psychiatric diagnosis of any individual offender. In this context it is not being suggested that criminal behavior can be construed as a formal mental disorder or psychiatric diagnosis in the way that some researchers such as Giannangelo *(26)*, for example, have argued. Rather, the present discussion is concerned with studying the pattern of constituent psychological characteristics that are commonly presented by serial criminals. It is from identifying the combination of these characteristics that their expression as behaviors at the scene of a crime can be taken to be indicative of a serial offender. In turn, these specific patterns of criminal behavior can be articulated as criteria in the definition of serial crime.

Psychopathy

Although serial offenders are seldom found to be legally insane *(27,28)*, among the various dimensions of personality that have been attributed to the serial sexual criminal are those that echo psychiatrically defined personality disorders. The dimension of psychopathy and the associated psychiatric diagnosis of antisocial personality disorder have attracted extensive consideration in this context *(29)*.

Psychopathy entails persistent violation of the rights of others, a disregard for such rights, a lack of empathy for the feelings of others, a lack of remorse for any offense or injury to others, an inflated self-concept, and superficial charm *(30)*. According to analyses of case material *(31–33)* and a few psychometric studies *(29)*, some behaviors of serial criminals are marked by such characteristics.

An act of murder, rape, or arson clearly constitutes a violation of another person's rights. But the acts of the serial criminal are frequently callous in the extreme, a cardinal feature of psychopathy *(34)*. The victim of a serial murderer or serial rapist is not simply killed or sexually penetrated but is typically used as an object of perverse gratification; various forms of torture are very common, as is postmortem mutilation of the victim's body *(6)*. Also highly characteristic of the serial offender is a lack of shame and remorse for the crimes committed and an evident immunity to the feelings of the victim, although the serial criminal may be so manipulative that a repentant posture may be assumed if it is potentially advantageous. Psychopathic manipulativeness also is evident in some serial criminals' use of superficial charm to lure a potential victim away from safety *(20)*.

Although there certainly is scope for more precise psychometric studies of the associations between specific features of psychopathy and specific features of serial sexual criminal behavior, it is fair to conclude there are strong indications that the personality dimension of psychopathy is often an element of the psychological profile of the serial offender.

This conclusion should not be taken as an unqualified endorsement of the popular depiction of the serial criminal as a quintessential psychopath. As Geberth and Turco *(31)* note, not all psychopaths will commit violent crimes, and not all serial offenders will meet the diagnostic criteria for antisocial personality disorder. A few behaviors of serial sexual offenders are in fact uncharacteristic of psychopathy.

Whereas psychopaths typically are impulsive and do not plan their activities thoroughly *(35)*, a substantial proportion of serial criminals are organized and methodical in the commission of their crimes *(11)*. The psychopath's renowned lack of empathy for the feelings of others also provides only a simplistic interpretation of the serial offender's lack of concern for the impact of their actions on others; after all, if a serial offender aims to terrorize, humiliate, dominate, and inflict extreme suffering on a victim *(31)*, some degree of empathy is necessary for the offender's appreciation of the degree of their success. Similarly, the irresponsibility of many psychopaths should not be overgeneralized as applying to all serial offenders because instances are clearly available of serial sexual murderers who, for example, were regarded as reliable and conscientious workers *(18,36)*. Although psychopathy is a significant element of the serial offender's psychological makeup, some account must also be taken of other dimensions of personality.

Narcissism

A personality dimension sometimes found in association with psychopathy is pathological narcissism. In simple terms, narcissism entails a concentration of psychological interest in the self *(37)*. Of course, a degree of self-interest is essential to healthy functioning, but at pathological levels narcissism presents as a pervasive pattern of grandiosity, need for admiration, and lack of empathy *(34)*. The narcissist's exaggerated self-esteem nevertheless is very fragile, and thus the person must periodically make rather grandiose efforts to buttress the narcissistic defenses and the self-image.

Relatively little research effort has been devoted to the identification of narcissistic tendencies in serial criminals, perhaps because narcissism does not share the notoriety associated with psychopathy. Nonetheless, specific features used for the differential diagnosis of pathological narcissism *(34)* can be recognized in the behaviors of individual serial offenders.

Like psychopathy, narcissism entails a lack of empathy for others. But whereas the psychopath simply sees other people as objects for self-gratification, narcissists need to establish a sense of superiority over others and demand admiration from others *(34)*. This aspect of narcissism is evident in many serial sexual offenders. Thus, Ritter *(32)* reports episodic murderers as exhibiting egocentrism and feelings of superiority and dominance. In individual case studies, serial offenders are often reported as having expressed both their own perceived superiority over their victims and a demeaning perception of their victims as less than human and thus deserving the violations perpetrated on them. Similarly, many serial offenders are said to have declared their intellectual superiority over police pursuing them and have even derided the competence of investigators *(38)*. Some serial offenders also claim to have allowed themselves to be apprehended, or to have intentionally left clues at a crime scene to ensure that investigative efforts of police continue to be focused on them *(22,39)*.

The precarious self-esteem or ego structure of narcissists also can be found in serial criminals. When circumstances challenge the narcissist's feelings of superiority, action, for example, flight, is necessary in order to reintegrate or re-establish their sense of superiority. The same pattern of behavior can be seen in the pre-crime stressors that set off the serial offender to commit crimes. As Hickey *(8)* reports, interviews with serial offenders have documented the periodic experience of feeling low followed by an outbreak of violent behavior to rebuild the sense of dominance and superiority. In the view of Geberth *"A serial killer, despite his outward facade, is a very insecure individual. He is without any power until he has a victim under his control"* (*4*, p. 47).

Another example of this fallible ego structure may be found in serial offenders' experience of considerable shock and disbelief when they are unexpectedly apprehended. In this disintegrated state they sometimes confess to their offenses. Later, when they re-integrate their ego, they may recant their confession, insisting it was a result of duress *(40)*.

A narcissistic need for admiration may underpin some of the exhibitionistic behaviors of serial offenders. Australian serial murderer John Glover, for example, assumed an air of intellectual authority, often boasting of his acumen despite never having pursued any form of tertiary education *(18)*. North American serial murderer Edmund Kemper readily cooperated with police investigators in locating incriminating evidence when he was given the impression of being in command of the investigation. According to Ressler and Shachtman *(22)*, the more praise Kemper received for the ingenuity of his offenses, the more information he revealed. Therefore, characteristics of pathological narcissism can be seen in the behavior of some serial offenders. It must be stressed, however, that there seem to be very few adequate psychometric studies undertaken on this issue. Additionally, aggression and deceit are behaviors that are specifically nominated as uncharacteristic of narcissists *(34)*, yet these clearly are prominent attributes of many serial criminals. The psychological features of the serial offender therefore encompasses elements of both psychopathy and narcissism.

Sadism

Sadism is characterized by a pervasive pattern of cruel, demeaning, and aggressive behavior *(41)*. Sadists take pleasure in the psychological or physical suffering of others. Psychopathy is sometimes associated with sadism, but conceptually and diagnostically these two personality dimensions can be distinguished. For example, although sadists are aggressive and brutalizing, they usually do not act in an illegal or socially unacceptable manner. Also, not all sadists inflict pain through physical violence, emotional abuse, and humiliation *(41)*.

Almost invariably, the crimes committed by serial murderers and rapists are sadistic. Violence is used not merely as a means of subduing the victim, but more fundamentally a source of pleasure for the offender. The serial criminal seeks to terrorize, demean, and humiliate the victim. As noted previously, acts of torture often are involved *(6)*. Similarly, most serial murders are committed in a distinctly personalized manner involving "skin-to-skin" contact between the victim and the offender (e.g., as in strangulation or stabbing); such "impersonal" methods of murder, such as poisoning, are infrequently observed among serial offenders.

The means of disposing of a victim's corpse can also be taken to suggest an offender's intent to humiliate and degrade. Rather than disposing of a corpse in a secretive location to avoid detection, the corpse might be purposely dumped in an open location where it is certain to be seen by others. Further, a corpse may be posed in a degrading or dramatic position intended to shock observers and thereby further humiliate the deceased. An example of a similar behavior in rape is the intentional release of a nude victim *(42)* or defecation in a burnt structure in the circumstance of arson.

Sadists are further described as inclined to restrict the autonomy of people with whom they hold a close relationship. This behavior often is observed in serial offenders who have a spouse. Such domination is reported to have sometimes reached the point in which partners have become slaves and assistants to the commission of crimes *(43)*.

Retrospective investigation of the childhood and adolescence of serial murderers *(11,22)* suggests that these sadistic tendencies develop well before the commission of the serial offenses. In childhood, these offenders' sadistic acts appear initially to have been directed at animals, and subsequently at peers. Furthermore, as children these offenders were frequently both victims and observers of violence.

Although the personality dimensions of psychopathy, narcissism, and sadism are diagnostically distinct, they seemingly function in a coherent, interactive fashion in the psychological make-up of the serial offender. Broadly speaking, psychopathy frees the offender from the injunctions of society against narcissistic and sadistic behavior; narcissism defines the primacy of self-gratification in the offender's lifestyle and fuels the sense of superiority by which the offender self-justifies sadistic and psychopathic behavior; and sadism gives form to the antisocial self-gratification and pursuit of superiority and dominance.

Kernberg *(44,45)* proposed an interesting concept that integrates these elements. Kernberg describes malignant narcissism as an extreme form of antisocial personality disorder that is manifest in a person who is pathologically grandiose, lacking in conscience and behavioral regulation, and with characteristic demonstrations of joyful cruelty and sadism *(46)*. The potential relevance of malignant narcissism to an understanding of serial violent crime has been suggested by Pollock *(46)*, but to date the joint problems of operationalizing and measuring malignant narcissism seem to have hampered any direct empirical investigation of the concept *(31)*. Additionally, the notion of malignant narcissism would seem not to give due acknowledgment to the role of psychosexual factors in serial crime.

Paraphilic Tendencies

Direct evidence of the role of sexual gratification in serial crime is difficult to identify and define. The involvement of sexual behavior in serial rape is obvious, but that the motivation of such behavior is necessarily more sexual than sadistic or narcissistic, for example, is unclear. Nonetheless, less direct support for the significance of sexual motives in a serial offender's psychological make-up is provided by reports of sexual behaviors performed in conjunction with these crimes and, more generally, serial offenders' deviant sexual tendencies.

Paraphilias are enduring patterns of sexual behavior in which unusual objects, rituals, or situations appear to be necessary for the person's full sexual satisfaction *(35)*. Often, these paraphilic behaviors have a compulsive quality. There is substantial literature documenting the occurrence of paraphilic behavior during the commission of serial crime. Sexual sadism or excitement obtained by inflicting physical or psychological pain on another person is an extremely common component of serial sexual murder. Reported examples include partially or completely disrobing the victim, the purposeful wounding and mutilation of a victim's breasts or genitalia, evidence of offender masturbation at the scene, or insertion of objects into the victim's anal or vaginal cavity *(11)*.

Fetishism, or the need for specific inanimate objects in sexual gratification, also seems to be involved in some cases of serial murder and serial rape. Thus, a serial offender may target victims who wear red high-heeled shoes or who have long dark hair, for example. Similarly, souvenirs of the crime may be taken by the offender not only to assist in reminiscing about the crime, but also for use in sexual fantasies *(11,47)*. The psychosexual function of serial offenders' souvenir collections is consistent with the fact that taking souvenirs is not common in other forms of crime, presumably because the discovery of such material by police provides a link to an offense that may prove highly incriminating.

Other aspects of a serial crime may serve a paraphilic function. Stab wounds inflicted on a victim's body might well be inspired in part by sadism, but they could simultaneously be sexually satisfying to the offender, representing a type of penetration. Indeed, such wounds are often found to be inflicted near the victim's genitals or breasts *(48)*. Picquerism, which is an intense desire to stab, wound, or cut the flesh of another person, is in fact a recognized (albeit rare) paraphilia. At times, pedophilia is also apparent in victim selection as illustrated by a number of cases, including American serial murderers John Gacy and Albert Fish *(40,49)*. Other paraphilias possibly associated with the commission of a serial sexual crime include flagellation (sexual excitement obtained by beating, whipping, or clubbing another person), necrophilia (a sexual attraction to dead bodies), and anthropophagi (sexual excitement from eating human flesh) *(50–53)*.

The psychosexual dimension of serial crime is often supported by evidence of the offender's masturbation at the scene of their crimes. Although not commonly associated with serial rape, evidence of masturbation is frequently found in serial murders and arsons *(20,54)*. Although autoerotic stimulation in this context may serve several functions (including defilement of the victim), its occurrence is consistent with the view that sexual stimulation or excitation may be derived through the commission of some crimes. Masturbation at the scene of serial arson offenses also confirms the view that serial arson might not be simply a property crime; rather, there is an important class of serial arson that is motivated by psychosexual factors *(55–57)*.

Paraphilic behavior outside the context of the crime also is common among serial offenders, suggesting that psychosexual dynamics play a central role in the offender's life. Serial murderers are reported to show a very high incidence of voyeurism, exhibitionism, fetishism, sadomasochism, frotteurism, coprophilia, bestiality, and pornography use *(58,59)*.

There are clear indications, therefore, that the form of self-gratification derived from the commission of serial crime is governed not only by sadism, but also by psychosexual motives. Again, paraphilic tendencies are presumed to function in an interactive way with psychopathy, narcissism, and sadism in the psychological make-up of the serial offender.

Fantasy Proneness and Dissociative Tendencies

As noted previously, serial offenders are seldom found to be legally insane *(27,28)*; that is, it is usually the case that at the time of the commission of their crimes, serial offenders were in control of what they were doing and knew that what they were doing was wrong. For many people, this fact makes it difficult to comprehend how the serial offender would be able to commit such callous and brutal acts. As previously discussed, part of the answer to this circumstance lies in the psychopathic, narcissistic, and sadistic psychology of the serial offender; however, there is more to it than this. The concept of legal sanity does not mean that the reality of the crime in the eyes of an objective observer was the reality experienced at the time by the offender. Understanding the serial criminal therefore requires an appreciation of the aberrant subjective reality in which such an offender operates.

In some instances, the subjective reality of the serial offender is unequivocally psychotic. That is, although still being in control of their actions, some serial criminals are driven to perceive the world in a deluded way, and this delusion inspires them to criminal action. For example, North American serial murderer Richard Trenton Chase killed victims to drink their blood, believing it would prevent his own blood from evaporating *(60)*. Edward Gein skinned corpses to construct masks and clothing in the belief that wearing such articles would transform him into another person *(22)*. Although such cases are relatively uncommon *(27,28,61,62)*, they draw attention to a crucial feature of serial crime: that such offenses are grounded in the aberrant fantasy world of the serial criminal.

Fantasy proneness is a personality characteristic entailing a persistent pattern of deep involvement in fantasy and imagination *(63)*. The fantasy-prone individual spends much of his or her waking life in fantasy, and the imaginative involvement is so intense that the experience of fantasy is extremely vivid and realistic. Fantasy-prone people tend to have a history of severe childhood abuse and emotional isolation *(63)*.

Although direct psychometric data are lacking, there are anecdotal indications that serial offenders may tend to be highly fantasy prone. For example, Hickey (*8*, p. 95) discusses possible elements of violent fantasy being emulated in the behavior of the serial killer Jeffrey Dahmer. Sexually violent serial offenders are reported to be preoccupied with sexually sadistic fantasies involving ritualized behavior *(8,58,64)*. The repeated, stylized patterns observed in the crime scenes of serial sexual offenders also point to the pivotal role of fantasy in these crimes. Certainly the *modus operandi* of serial offenses may adapt and change as the offender becomes more experienced, but according to Douglas and Munn *(65)*, the fantasy scenario that drives these behaviors is static and remains constant in each offense. In effect, the underlying fantasy represents the serial offender's signature. Stoller *(66)* and Drukteinis *(67)* have both speculated that the psychological function of this fantasy is to convert memories of childhood trauma into a sense of control and mastery over life. Hickey *(8)* further speculates on the role of violent fantasies as being an instrumental component in creating the psychological drive to commit further offenses.

The posited role of fantasy in serial crime also helps explain one of the distinctive features of such crime: the choice of strangers as victims. In most conventional murders, rapes, or arsons some form of prior relationship will exist between the victim and offender, and this relationship provides a key motive for the offense *(5)*. In serial sexual crimes, however, the motive is the underlying fantasy with which the offender is preoccupied. A prior relationship between the victim and the offender therefore need not, and typically does not, exist. What is important is the role that the victim represents in the offender's fantasy.

The serial offender's deep absorption in fantasy signals the significance of a personality dimension closely related to fantasy proneness: dissociative tendencies. Dissociation entails a separation between cognitive processes that ordinarily would be linked. In the dissociative state of highway hypnosis, for example, a driver may be deeply engrossed in thought and seemingly oblivious to road conditions, yet the car remains on the road; here, the cognitive processes involved in navigating the road are temporarily separated or dissociated from the conscious involvement in thought. The driver still knows what he or she is doing with the car and still owns the responsibility for the driving behavior. An exacerbation of dissociative tendencies has been linked to a history of childhood trauma *(68)*.

There are at least some anecdotal indications of dissociative processes among serial criminals *(8,69)*. During the commission of the crime a serial offender may perceive the victim as a mere object, something less than human. This process of dehumanization may be dissociative; the offender knows the victim is a sentient being but dissociates this knowledge while treating the victim as an object for use in self-gratification. Conversely, when victims have engaged an offender in personal conversation to develop rapport, this has, at times, impeded the offender's ability to dissociate the victim's humanness, resulting in some victims escaping with their lives *(8,39,70)*.

Further, in some instances, serial offenders have described their state of mind during the commission of their offenses as dreamlike, akin to the state of highway hypnosis discussed earlier. Although the sincerity of offenders' accounts cannot be viewed uncritically, surviving victims of some serial offenders have described their attacker as in a trance-like state, devoid of emotion, and glassy-eyed *(39)*. Admittedly, in some instances offenders seek to facilitate the process of dissociation by using psychotropic substances such as alcohol *(8,11)*.

Again, the dissociative quality of offenders' experience of their crimes is consistent with the fact that some of these recollections are described in the third person *(71)*. If serial offenders rely on dissociation, these defenses are likely to be used not only during the crime, but afterwards as well. Awareness of the sentient nature of the victim and of the more gory aspects of an assault may have to be dissociated from the offender's other memories of the crime. Furthermore, it is possible that the fantasy driving the serial offender is a dissociated expression of a pathological need for control induced by a history of childhood trauma *(11,67)*.

The possibility that serial criminals qualify for the psychiatric diagnosis of a dissociative disorder such as dissociative identity (multiple personality) disorder continues to be a contentious issue, and certainly there have been cases in which such a claim was advanced in a mischievous endeavor to avoid conviction *(72)*. The proposed dissociative tendencies of serial offenders also await appropriate psychometric investigation. The incorporation of dissociative tendencies into the make-up of the serial offender nevertheless seems to illuminate some aspects of the behavior of these offenders.

Therefore, the cognitive processes associated with the psychopathic, narcissistic, sadistic, and paraphilic elements of serial crime are proposed to be strongly marked by fantasy and dissociation. Nonetheless, serial offenders' heavy involvement in fantasy should not be taken to imply that offenses are necessarily out of all touch with reality. Here, fantasy is imposed on reality; it is the script that is acted out at the scene of the crime, engaging the victim as an unwilling but leading player. Except perhaps in rare psychotic cases, the directors of the dramatic production appreciate their actions.

Compulsiveness

A seemingly obvious and yet often unacknowledged mechanism in serial offenders is their compulsive drive to re-offend. In contrast to mass or spree offenders who offend in a single burst, serial offenders are distinguished by their intermittent pattern of offenses.

Several researchers have documented a characteristic cycle in the behavior of serial offenders *(8,11,73)*. This cycle starts with the offender experiencing a growing sense of tension marked by increasingly intense sadistic and paraphilic fantasies. The tension gradually accumulates until it seemingly compels the commission of an offense, which in turn acts as a release for the tension. Following the crime, there is a "cooling off" period in which the offender experiences a temporary state of relaxation. However, the relaxation soon dissipates, and the cycle resumes with another build-up of tension. The offender seems unable to resist the compulsion of the cycle, and therefore re-offends. The length of the intermissions between offenses, however, is not constant either within or between offenders.

This feature of compulsiveness in serial offenders has not received due attention from researchers. Possibly the compulsiveness has a physiological basis. Simon *(73)* remarked on the similarity of the serial offense cycle to that associated with substance abuse. On these grounds, Simon hypothesized that the etiology of serial crime entails some form of physiological addiction. It may be noted that the addiction model of serial crime is consistent with some physiological and neurochemical data obtained from serial murderers *(74)*.

Although further empirical investigation is clearly warranted, compulsiveness is nominated as an important facet of the psychological make-up of the serial criminal. Specifically, the fantasy underlying the offender's crime pattern is so engrossing to them that it is irresistible, driving the offender to commit an interminable succession of offenses without ever reaching a state of final satiation.

CONCLUSION

This chapter argues that the term serial crime signifies not so much a series of similar offenses *per se*, but rather a psychological propensity to commit a series of similar offenses. Analysis of the psychological characteristics of serial sexual offenders indeed suggests that there are coherent psychological mechanisms associated with serial sexual crime. The psychological make-up canvassed in this chapter traces the serial criminal's psychological propensity to re-offend in a consistent fashion.

A review of the existing literature concerning the predominant psychological characteristics of serial criminals discussed herein provides a coherent account of the psychodynamics of their crimes to the extent that a discrete psychological make-up emerges. The serial offender is marked by a distinctive complex mix of psychopathic, narcissistic, sadistic, paraphilic, and fantasy-prone tendencies. Psychopathy frees the offender from the injunctions of society against narcissistic and sadistic behavior. Narcissism defines the primacy of self-gratification in the offender's lifestyle and fuels the sense of superiority by which the offender self-justifies sadistic and psychopathic behavior. Both sadism and paraphilic tendencies give form to the antisocial self-gratification and pursuit of superiority and dominance. The psychopathic, narcissistic, sadistic, and paraphilic dynamics are integrated into a compulsive fantasy that governs the offender's style of victimization and also allows the offender to dissociate from aspects of the criminal act that would detract from the enactment of the fantasy. The offender's impelling fantasy has a virtually addictive quality, cycling through a progressively increasing compulsion to enact the fantasy, the achievement of temporary satiety through commission of the offense, and a period of respite before the fantasy begins to take hold once more.

This chapter argues that serial crime can be defined as an offense in which the style of victimization is consistent with the psychological make-up, that is, one marked by a compulsive criminal fantasy with psychopathic, narcissistic, sadistic, and paraphilic elements. The serial style of victimization may become evident through (a) crime scene data and witness reports concerning a single offense, (b) piecing together crime scene data and witness reports over a series of offenses, or (c) less frequently, the confessions of the offender.

Table 5.1 presents distinctive characteristics of the serial style of victimization that may be observed in cases of serial/sexual murder, rape, and arson. These characteristics are identified as direct behavioral expressions of

Table 5.1
Indicators of Serial Violent Style of Victimisation

Murder

- Postmortem mutilation of the corpse (e.g., evisceration, dismemberment, cannibalism)
- Intentionally stylized and/or dramatic positioning of corpse
- Sexual assault (e.g., rape) of victim
- Necrophilic activity with corpse or body parts
- Injuries in excess of those required to effect victim's death
- Pre-mortem torture
- Souvenir collection (e.g., victim's garments, body parts)

Rape

- Stylized vocal scripts demanded from the victim
- Sadistic/violent treatment of victim (e.g., disrobing, torture, biting, beating)
- Other paraphilic activities with victim (e.g., digital manipulation, sodomy, urogalia)
- Offender's failure or inability to penetrate victim or to climax
- Souvenir collection (e.g., victim's garments or personal effects)

Arson

- Destruction of property in addition to fire damage
- Sexual activity at crime scene (e.g., masturbation)
- Offender's "signature" intentionally left at crime scene (e.g., graffiti, fecal matter)
- Intentional stylized activity either in fire initiation or in other activities at crime scene

the psychopathic, narcissistic, sadistic, and paraphilic tendencies inherent in the criminal fantasy of the serial offender. Note that in each instance the behaviors constitute activity far in excess of what would be required simply to kill a victim, to sexually penetrate a victim, or to ignite an object.

The behaviors listed in Table 5.1, however, are a preliminary approximation of the serial sexual style of victimization and are by no means exhaustive of the behaviors that may be observed. Two matters warrant clarification. First, the serial style of victimization takes no account of the number of offenders. It is assumed that a serial violent crime with multiple offenders will entail either the collaboration of individuals who possess the defining psychological make-up, and/or the domination of a subservient partner by a person who has the posited make-up. Although some offender taxonomies distinguish serial crimes perpetrated by an individual from those perpetrated by multiple offenders *(8)*, there seems no advantage in adopting such a distinction. Second, although the present serial style of victimization focuses on the proneness of an offender to continue offending even if only a single offense has been committed, the behaviors listed in Table 5.1 are not intended as a measure for predicting recidivism in correctional settings or judicial matters.

The factors discussed in this chapter form the definition of serial violent crime and the sampling basis for a number of the CAP studies canvassed in subsequent chapters throughout this book. It is argued that it is the type of crimes fitting this definition that are most likely to benefit from the use of criminal profiling in a practical investigative context.

Acknowledgment

Material canvassed in this chapter has been revised from a previously published manuscript by: Kocsis, R.N. and Irwin, H.J. (1998). The psychological profile of serial offenders and a redefinition of the misonomer of serial crime. Psychiatry, Psychology and Law, 5(2), 197–213.

References

1. Salfati, C.G. (2000). The nature of expressiveness and instrumentality in homicide. Homicide Studies, 4(3), 265-293.
2. Daly, M. and Wilson, M. (1988). Homicide. New York: Aldine de Gruyter.
3. Polk, K. (1994). When men kill: Scenarios of masculine violence. Cambridge, UK: Cambridge University Press.
4. Geberth, V.J. (1986). The investigation of sex related homicides. Law and Order, 34(7), 40–48.
5. Geberth, V.J. (1986). Mass, serial and sensational homicides: The investigative perspective. Journal of Urban Health, 62, 492–496.
6. Douglas, J.E., Burgess, A.W., Burgess, A.G., Ressler, R.K. (1992). Crime classification manual. New York: Simon & Schuster.
7. Holmes, R.M. and Holmes, S.T. (1998). Serial murder, 2nd ed. Newbury Park, CA: Sage.
8. Hickey, E.W. (1997). Serial murderers and their victims, 2nd ed. Fresno, CA: Wadsworth.
9. Brooks, P., Devine, M., Green, T., Hart, B., Moore, M. (1988). Serial murder: A criminal justice response. Police Chief, 54(6), 37–45.
10. Canter, D. and Larkin, P. (1993). The environmental range of serial rapists. Journal of Environmental Psychology, 13, 63–69.
11. Ressler, R.K., Burgess, A., Douglas, J.E. (1988). Sexual homicide: Patterns and motives. New York: Lexington Books.
12. Hickey, E.W. (1990). Serial murderers and their victims. Fresno, CA: Wadsworth.
13. Fox, J.A. and Levin, J. (1994). Overkill: Mass murder and serial killing exposed. New York: Plenum Press.
14. Levin, J. and Fox, J.A. (1985). Mass murder: America's growing menace. New York: Plenum Press.

15. Leyton, E. (1986). Compulsive killers: The story of modern multiple murder. New York: New York University Press.
16. Norris, J. (1988). Serial killers: The growing menace. New York: Doubleday.
17. Rappaport, R.G. (1988). The serial and mass murderer: Patterns, differentiation, pathology. American Journal of Forensic Psychiatry, 9, 39–48.
18. Simpson, L. and Harvey, S. (1994). The killer next door: Death in an Australian suburb. Sydney: Random House.
19. Writer, L., Barrett, S., Bouda, S. (1992). Garden of evil: The granny killer's reign of terror. Sydney: Ironbark Press.
20. Rule, A. (1989). The stranger beside me. London: Warner.
21. Wilkes, G.A. and Krebs, W.A. (1992). Collin's English dictionary, 3rd ed. Sydney: Harper Collins.
22. Ressler, R.K. and Shachtman, T. (1992). Whoever fights monsters. London: Simon & Schuster.
23. Jenkins, P. (1993). Chance or choice: The selection of serial murder victims. In: Wilson, A.V., ed. Homicide: The victim/offender connection. Cincinnati, OH: Anderson, pp. 461–477.
24. Wilson, P.R. (1985). Murder of the innocents: Child killers and their victims. Singapore: Rigby.
25. McGregor, A. (1990). Murdered innocence. Australian Police Journal, 44, 145–154.
26. Giannangelo, S.J. (1996). The psychopathology of serial murder: A theory of violence. London: Praeger.
27. Brown, J.S. (1991). The psychopathology of serial sexual homicide: A review of the possibilities. American Journal of Forensic Psychiatry, 12, 13–21.
28. Palermo, G.B. and Knudten, R.D. (1994). The insanity plea in the case of a serial killer. International Journal of Offender Therapy and Comparative Criminology, 38, 3–16.
29. Blackburn, R. (1993). The psychology of criminal conduct: Theory, research and practice. Chichester, UK: Wiley.
30. Cleckley, H. (1988). The mask of sanity, 5th ed. Augusta, GA: Mosby.
31. Geberth, V.J. and Turco, R.N. (1997). Antisocial personality disorder, sexual sadism, malignant narcissism, and serial murder. Journal of Forensic Science, 42, 49–60.
32. Ritter, B.J. (1989). Multiple murderers: The characteristics of the persons and the nature of their crimes (Doctoral dissertation, United States International University, 1988). Dissertation Abstracts International, 49A, 1971–1972.
33. Stone, M.H. (1993). Abnormalities of personality: Within and beyond the realm of treatment. New York: Norton.
34. Kocsis, R. N., Cooksey, R. W., Irwin, H. J. (2002). Psychological profiling of sexual murders: An empirical model. International Journal of Offender Therapy and Comparative Criminology, 46(3), 532–553.
35. American Psychiatric Association. (1994). Diagnostic and statistical manual of mental disorders, 4th ed. Washington, DC: Author.
36. Shears, R. (1996). Highway to nowhere. Sydney: Harper Collins.
37. Wink, P. (1996). Narcissism. In: Costello, C.G., ed. Personality characteristics of the personality disordered. New York: Wiley, pp. 146–172.
38. Hazelwood, R.R., Dietz, P.E., Warren, J. (1992). The criminal sexual sadist. FBI Law Enforcement Bulletin, 61(2), 12–20.

39. Douglas, J.E. and Olshaker, M. (1995). Mindhunter. New York: Scribner.
40. Cahill, T. (1986). Buried dreams: Inside the mind of a serial killer. New York: Bantam Books.
41. American Psychiatric Association. (1987). Diagnostic and statistical manual of mental disorders, 3rd ed., rev. Washington, DC: Author.
42. Geberth, V.J. (1995). The signature aspects in criminal investigation: Criminal personality profiling. Law and Order, 43(11), 45–49.
43. Hazelwood, R.R., Warren, J., Dietz, P.E. (1993). Compliant victims of the sexual sadist. Australian Family Physician, 22, 474–479.
44. Kernberg, O.F. (1984). Aggression in personality disorders and perversions. New Haven, CT: Yale University Press.
45. Kernberg, O.F. (1992). Severe personality disorders. New Haven, CT: Yale University Press.
46. Pollock, P.H. (1995). A case of spree serial murder with suggested diagnostic opinions. International Journal of Offender Therapy and Comparative Criminology, 39, 258–267.
47. Singh, C.A. (1993). A psychological profile of serial murderers involved in trophy collection. Unpublished master's thesis, California State University, Fresno, CA.
48. DeRiver, J. (1956). The sexual criminal. Springfield, IL: C.C. Thomas.
49. Lane, B. and Gregg, W. (1992). The encyclopaedia of serial killers. London: Headline.
50. Fahy, T.A., Wessely, S., David, A. (1988). Werewolves, vampires and cannibals. Medicine, Science, and Law, 28, 145–149.
51. Kayton, L. (1972). The relationship of the vampire legend to schizophrenia. Journal of Youth and Adolescence, 1, 303–314.
52. Prins, H. (1984). Vampirism: Legendary or clinical phenomenon? Medicine, Science, and Law, 24, 283–293.
53. Prins, H. (1985). Vampirism: A clinical condition. British Journal of Psychiatry, 146, 666–668.
54. Frank, G. (1966). The Boston strangler. New York: New American Library.
55. Geller, J.L. (1987). Firesetting in the adult psychiatric population. Hospital and Community Psychiatry, 38, 501–506.
56. Geller, J.L. (1992). Arson in review: From profit to pathology. Psychiatric Clinics of North America, 15, 623–645.
57. Geller, J.L. (1992). Pathological fire-setting in adults. International Journal of Law Psychiatry, 15, 283–302.
58. Prentky, R.A., Burgess, A.W., Rokous, F., et al. (1989). The presumptive role of fantasy in serial sexual homicide. American Journal of Psychiatry, 146, 887–891.
59. Ressler, R.K., Burgess, A.W., Douglas, J.E., Hartman, C.R., D'Agostino, R.B. (1986). Sexual killers and their victims: Identifying patterns through crime scene analysis. Journal of Interpersonal Violence, 1, 288–308.
60. Biondi, R. and Hecox, W. (1992). The Dracula killer. New York: Simon & Schuster.
61. Bourguignon, A. (1982). Vampirism and autovampirism. In: Schlesinger, L.B. and Revitch, E., eds. Sexual dynamics of antisocial behavior. Springfield, IL: Thomas, pp. 37–62.

62. Dietz, P.E. (1986). Mass, serial and sensational homicides. Journal of Urban Health, 62, 477–491.
63. Lynn, S.J. and Rhue, J.W. (1988). Fantasy proneness: Hypnosis, developmental antecedents, and psychopathology. American Psychologist, 43, 35–44.
64. Ressler, R.K., Burgess, A., Douglas, J.E., Hazelwood, R.R. (1985). Interviewing techniques for sexual homicide investigation. FBI Law Enforcement Bulletin, 54(8), 26–32.
65. Douglas, J.E. and Munn, C. (1992). Violent crime scene analysis: Modus operandi, signature and staging. FBI Law Enforcement Bulletin, 61(2), 1–10.
66. Stoller, R.E. (1975). Perversion. New York: Pantheon Books.
67. Drukteinis, A.M. (1992). Serial murder: The heart of darkness. Psychiatric Annals, 22, 532–538.
68. Irwin, H.J. (1994). Proneness to dissociation and traumatic childhood events. Journal of Nervous and Mental Disease, 182, 456–460.
69. Vetter, H. (1992). Dissociation, psychopathy, and the serial murderer. In: Egger, S.A., ed. Serial murder: An elusive phenomenon. New York: Praeger, pp. 73–92.
70. Davis, D. (1991). The Milwaukee murders. New York: St. Marins.
71. Tanay, E. (1976). The murderers. Indianapolis: Bobbs-Merril.
72. Behnke, S.H. (1997). Confusion in the courtroom: How judges have assessed the criminal responsibility of individuals with multiple personality disorder. International Journal of Law Psychiatry, 20, 293–310.
73. Burgess, A.W., Hartman, C.R., Ressler, R.K., Douglas, J.E., McCormack, A. (1986). Sexual homicide: A motivational model. Journal of Interpersonal Violence, 1, 251–272.
74. Norris, J. (1988). Serial killers: The growing menace. New York: Doubleday.

Chapter 6

Operational Interpretation of the CAP Models

Summary

The research of Crime Action Profiling (CAP) is characterized by a set of distinct methodological procedures that have been used to develop models of crime behaviors and associated offender characteristics. The application of these models for profiling violent crimes can be achieved at a theoretically complex or simple, more practical level. The theoretical use of the CAP models predominantly involves an understanding of the methodological development of the models, the discernment of behavioral clusters, and the relevance they hold with previously proposed taxonomies of serial violent offenders. However, a less theoretically oriented application of the CAP models can also be achieved by those unfamiliar with complex statistical methodologies. Consequently, this chapter explains a set of generic principles whereby any of the CAP models can be interpreted for the purpose of developing a criminal profile without a detailed understanding of the methodologies inherent to the development of these models.

Key Words: CAP models; operational interpretation; criminal profiles.

Introduction

At the time of this book's publication, three major studies following the approach of Crime Action Profiling (CAP) have been developed for crimes of serial/sexual murder, serial rape, and serial arson. The findings of each study and specifically the diagrams generated therein can be used at a theoretically complex or simple, practical level. The theoretical perspective is predominately concerned with explaining the methodological principles involved in the development of the models, the identification of coherent behavioral clusters, and their compared similarity to typologies identified by other research-

From: *Criminal Profiling: Principles and Practice*
By: R. N. Kocsis © Humana Press Inc., Totowa, NJ

ers for serial violent crimes and offenders. On a more practical level, the same material and in particular the developed diagrams/models can also be interpreted to assist in the development of a criminal profile. Whereas Chapters 7–9 focus on the more complex theoretical exposition, the present chapter is dedicated to explaining how the CAP models can function on a simpler level. It should be noted that although the studies in the three subsequent chapters consider differing forms of violent crime, they all share the same methodological basis that characterizes the CAP approach to the profiling of these types of crimes. Consequently, the material that follows endeavors to provide a generic and easily comprehensible method by which a lay person unfamiliar with research methodologies and/or statistical procedures can nonetheless interpret the CAP models and apply them for the purpose of developing a criminal profile.

Understanding Multidimensional Scaling

Before explaining how to use any of the CAP models it is necessary to describe, to a limited extent, the statistical technique of multidimensional scaling (MDS) that is integral to the development of these models. At the outset it should be understood that MDS is not a method or technique for criminal profiling but merely a form of statistical analysis akin to other statistical measures, such as analysis of variance (ANOVA), for example. Additionally, it should be noted that MDS is not a statistic itself, but rather a type of statistical analysis. There are a number of different types of MDS that can be used to analyze different forms of data. A thorough explanation of MDS is simply not feasible within the scope of this book.* Instead, the objective of this section is to provide a lay person with an explanation, albeit rudimentary, of the general functions of MDS, that is, what MDS provides via the analysis of data.

Perhaps the best starting point in explaining MDS is to discuss the much simpler and somewhat similar statistical procedure of correlation. Imagine, for example, that one wishes to study the relationship, if any, between the sale of cold drinks and the daily temperature. In this hypothetical example we would be investigating the relationship, if any, between two variables: the number of drinks sold and the daily temperature. One method by which a scientist could investigate the relationship, if any, between these two variables would be to record the number of drinks sold over a number of days while also recording the corresponding temperature on each of those days. This daily recording of sales and temperature represents data that can be ana-

*Readers interested in a detailed explanation of MDS can refer to Coxon *(1)*.

lyzed using the statistical measure of correlation. A detailed understanding of the mathematical principles inherent to correlation is not necessary for the purposes of this discussion. Suffice to say that by incorporating the recorded data into a mathematical formula (which is the correlation statistic) some understanding of the relationship inherent to the data can be determined. The result of these calculations produces a number referred to in statistical parlance as a correlation coefficient. Depending on the size of this number as well as its polarity (i.e., whether the number is positive or negative), some understanding of the relationship between drink sales and temperature can be determined. Thus, in the hypothetical example the result of this statistical analysis provides a large positive number. In this circumstance we could conclude that a strong incremental relationship exists between the two variables. Interpreting this statistical result in the context of our example suggests that there is a tendency for drink sales to increase when the temperature rises. The hotter the day, the more drinks that are sold.

In some respects, MDS merely represents a more sophisticated form of correlation. That is, it is a statistical procedure that examines the relationships, if any, between variables. However, in explaining MDS there are two important features to bear in mind. First, in the previous example of correlation only two variables were considered, drink sales and temperature. MDS, however, is capable of simultaneously examining the relationships between numerous variables. The second important feature surrounding MDS is the method by which the results of the analysis concerning the relationships between variables are expressed. With correlation these relationships are communicated via the use of a number referred to as a correlation coefficient. However, the results of the statistical analysis derived from using MDS are typically depicted in the form of a diagram. These diagrams are predominantly structured in the shape of a large square that is referred to as a map in statistical parlance. For simplicity, however, in this discussion these MDS maps will simply be described as a diagram denoted by a large square. Within the square the differing variables that are the topic of the analysis are plotted via the use of small marks referred to as icons. It is the position of the icon within this square, relative to the position of any other icons (representing other variables) within the square that illustrates the relationship between the variables. Consequently, two icons representing two variables plotted on a MDS diagram in close proximity to each other indicates that these two variables hold a close or strong relationship to one another. A third icon located in a remote region of the square diagram relative to the position of the first two icons denotes that this third variable does not hold a strong, or possibly any relationship, with the first two.

In addition to conveying the relationship between individual variables their general location within the all-encompassing square also provides some indication, in one sense, of their commonality and/or frequency.* Icons depicted closer to the center of the square are more frequent and hold a common relationship to all variables. Conversely, icons located in the outlying regions of the square are more distinct and do not share many common relationships with the exception of other variables that may also be located in the same outlying region.

Possibly the best way to understand these concepts is by the use of a very simple hypothetical example. Imagine that a scientist wishes to study the differing types of motor vehicles. The first step in such a study would involve the development of a list of possible components found in motor vehicles. For the sake of simplicity, the list in this example will merely comprise of tires, carbon fiber chassis, steel chassis, steering wheel, and handlebars. Each of these items represents a separate variable in the scientist's study of motor vehicles. With this list of variables determined, a sample of motor vehicles would then need to be collected. Each of these vehicles would be examined to see which of the five variables on the list each particular vehicle featured. If a variable such as a carbon fiber chassis was observed to be present in the first vehicle then a value of 1 (for present) would be recorded. Similarly, if it was determined that this vehicle did not have a steering wheel then a value of 0 (for absent) would then be recorded. This recording of the presence or absence of each of these items inherent to each of the examined motor vehicles comprises the data for the scientist's study.

Given the mathematical complexity of MDS, most contemporary applications are achieved by using computer programs that perform the multitude of calculations inherent to this analysis and plot the results in the form of a diagram. Consequently, the data collected from our sample of motor vehicles would typically be entered into a computer program, which would then perform the analysis and generate a diagram representative of this analysis. Figure 6.1 represents a simplified MDS diagram using the hypothetical data of motor vehicles. It should be noted that the various arrows and dotted circles in Fig. 6.1 have been drawn in to assist with this basic explanation and do not actually represent part of the MDS diagram. Instead, the results of the analysis are contained in the large square outline within which are various spatial points

---

*As a somewhat technical qualification, this issue related to frequency is more applicable to MDS analysis of dichotomous data (i.e., 0 or 1 variables) such as that used in the CAP studies.

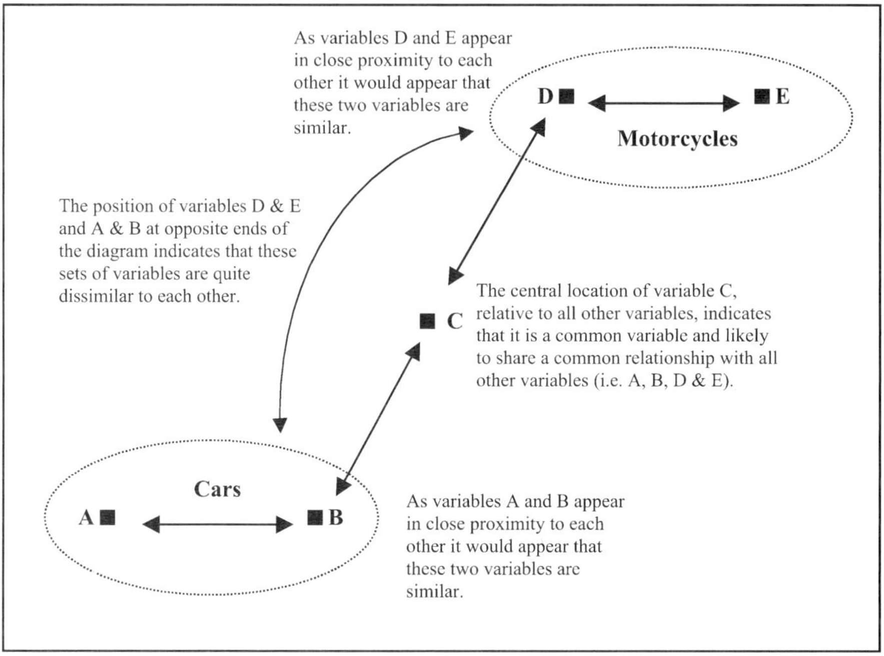

Fig. 6.1. Simplified multidimensional scaling diagram. **(A)**, steering wheel; **(B)**, steel chassis; **(C)**, tires; **(D)**, carbon fiber chassis; **(E)**, handlebars.

denoted by an icon. In this example, they appear in the shape of small black squares.

The icon representing tires is located in a position toward the center of the diagram. The central position of this icon indicates that tires are a commonly occurring feature in this analysis of motor vehicles and have a common relationship with all other variables in the diagram. Working outward, the diagram also depicts four other icons. First, the variable icons representative of a steering wheel and steel chassis are located close together in the bottom left corner of the diagram. Given their close proximity with one another it can be inferred that these two variables share a strong common relationship. Thus, an interpretation of the close proximity of these icons could be that motor vehicles that have a steering wheel are typically also likely to have a steel chassis. If one was to try and think of a description that reflects the features of the vehicles typically represented by these two variables, one could label them cars. Toward the top right corner of the MDS diagram, however, are the two variables of handlebars and carbon fiber chassis. Once again, the close proximity of these two variables to one another denotes a strong relationship between them. Akin to the previous description, a label that characterizes vehicles typically found to have these two variables could be motorcycles. Finally, given that the variables characteristic of both cars and motorcycles are located at opposite ends of the MDS diagram we could conclude that these two general types of motor vehicles are quite different from each other but they share the common feature of having tires as depicted by the tires icon located in a central position between them. By this example it is hoped that readers can see that MDS is a statistical procedure whereby coherent patterns in different variables can be identified and thus better understood.

It is in an analogous fashion that the CAP studies canvassed in Chapters 7–9 were undertaken. That is, in the circumstance of the sexual murder study in Chapter 8, for example, an extensive list of possible crime behaviors was first developed. This list represented the variables to be analyzed in the study. Next, a sample of actual sexual murder cases was collected. Each of these cases was then examined to ascertain the presence or absence of each of the variables and the results tabulated into data. This data was then analyzed using MDS to produce a diagram depicting the behavioral patterns observable in the commission of sexual murder offenses.

Linking Offender Characteristics

As discussed in the previous section, MDS represents a statistical tool for the analysis of data. The functional features of MDS are its ability to simultaneously analyze the relationships between numerous variables and communicate the results of this analysis via the use of a diagram. Consequently, one characteristic feature of the research methodology inherent to CAP is its analysis of crime behaviors using MDS. In this respect, Chapters 7–9 display the results of such analyses for large samples of sexual murderers, serial rapists, and serial arsonists. However, the use of MDS is only one methodological component inherent to the CAP models. That is, MDS only analyzes and allows for the identification of patterns in the studied crime behaviors. In effect, therefore, these MDS analyses only represent half of the profiling process in that it provides a method for interpreting crime behaviors. The other half of the process of criminal profiling involves discerning how any behavior patterns displayed in the MDS diagrams are related to offender characteristics.

The mathematical procedures inherent to the statistics used to achieve this goal are, once again, quite complex. Consequently, the objective of this section is not to explain the machinations of these procedures in developing the CAP models but rather to explain how the results of these analyses can be readily interpreted and applied. As previously discussed, each of the three studies contained in Chapters 7–9 involved collecting large samples of past cases involving sexual murder, serial rape, and serial arson, respectively. These cases provided the data for each of the studies. The process of analysis involved developing a list of crime behavior variables for the respective crimes, coding the presence or absence of these variables for each of the cases, and then using MDS to analyze the derived data for patterns and relationships. Concurrent to this analysis of the crime behaviors was another set of analyses on the characteristics of the apprehended offenders to each of the crimes. Thus, in a roughly similar fashion as the crime behaviors to each crime, a list, that is, a set of variables, was developed to describe all the possible attributes of the offenders for each crime. Examples of these variables included such characteristics as an offender's age, marital status, level of education, and so forth. The collected data concerning the offender's characteristics were then analyzed by comparing them to the data concerning the crime behaviors. Thus, akin to the earlier example of correlation, the data for the offender characteristics was analyzed using various statistical procedures to see which offender characteristics were, and were not, related to the various crime behaviors evident in the MDS diagrams.

It is the method by which the results of this analysis (i.e., the relationships between the crime behaviors and offender characteristics) are displayed that is one of the most distinctive methodological features of the CAP research. Indeed, it is this method of combining and displaying these two sets of analysis that forms the basis for referring to the products of these studies as **CAP models**. These relationships are displayed using large arrows that are orientated on a central point of axis and superimposed on top of the MDS diagram of the crime behavior patterns. At the end of each arrowhead is a set of offender characteristics or crime features.* These characteristics or crime features are linked with the particular arrow.

The process of interpreting the relationship between the characteristics listed at the point of each arrow and the crime behaviors is a reasonably straightforward process of looking at which arrows are positioned in the general proximity of a crime behavior icon located in the MDS diagram. One nuance incorporated into this matching process is that the arrows denote offender characteristics and crime features that are both related and unrelated to the crime behaviors depicted in the MDS diagram. This is determined from the position of the head and tail of each arrow. The head and the tail denote opposing polarities, that is, the presence or absence of a given characteristic.

*It should be noted that the term *crime features* is used because various types of information are examined beyond just the demographic features of offenders.

The offender characteristics for each arrow are always listed near the arrowhead. The characteristics that appear beside the arrowhead will be related to any crime behavior icons in the MDS diagram that are located in the proximity to that arrowhead. Conversely, crime behaviors that are located in proximity to the tail end of the same arrow in the same MDS diagram are unlikely to be related to the offender characteristics listed beside the arrow head.*

To better explain this process, Fig. 6.2 presents a simplified example of a CAP model. The model consists of the square MDS diagram that has been analyzed and therefore depicts crime behavior patterns. In this example, only a single arrow has been used and superimposed on top of the MDS diagram to demonstrate the process involved in interpreting the relationships between the variables. The arrow bisects the diagram from left to right with the arrowhead located in the upper right region of the square and the tail of the arrow located toward the lower left region of the square. The offender characteristics listed next to the arrowhead include offender vehicle, porn collection,† and white-collar job. The crime behaviors depicted in the general vicinity of the arrowhead in the MDS diagram are torture and gagged, indicating that these two behaviors are likely to be associated with offenders who possess a motor vehicle and a pornography collection and are employed in some type of white-collar job. This process of interpretation also operates in reverse. Because the arrow tail is located in the bottom left region of the MDS diagram near the crime behavior of postmortem sex, it can be surmised that these same offender characteristics will not be associated with this particular behavior. Thus, postmortem sexual activity at a crime scene is likely to be associated with an offender who **does not** possess a motor vehicle, a pornography collection, or have a white-collar job.

In conclusion, although the statistical procedures involved in developing the various CAP models are admittedly a little complex, the process of interpreting the models and thus understanding the relationships between crime behaviors and offender characteristics is relatively straightforward. Various arrows display a collection of offender characteristics. The proximate posi-

---

*The depiction of arrows was adjusted slightly in the CAP model on serial arsonists in Chapter 9. In this CAP model, the use of arrows was replaced with simple lines. These lines only point out towards offender/crime characteristic variables that hold a positive relationship (this is akin to the head of an arrow). However, these lines can also be used to interpret a negative relationship for the same offender/crime characteristic variables. This is accomplished by simply extending the same line in the opposite direction in the MDS diagram. This extension of the line in the opposite direction is akin to a tail of an arrow.

†An acronym for a pornography collection.

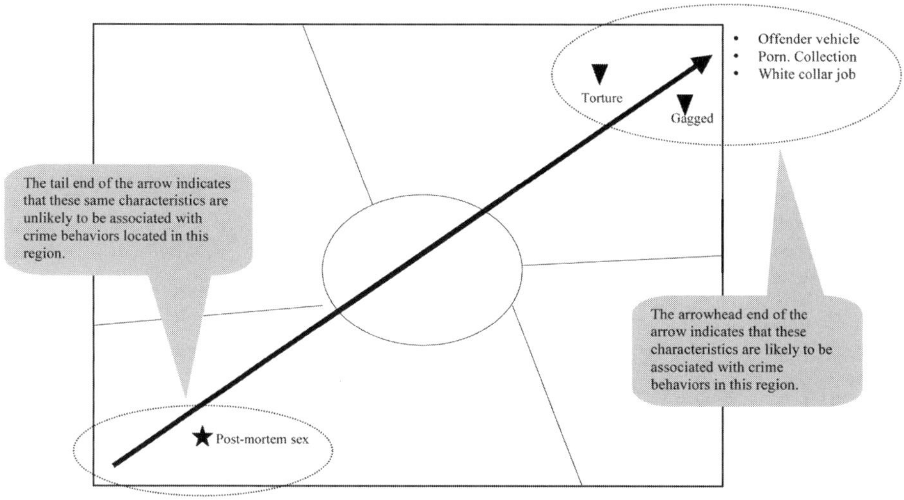

Fig. 6.2. A simplified example of a Crime Action Profiling model. The multidimensional scaling diagram depicts the patterns inherent to the various crime behaviors. The arrow superimposed on top illustrates the offender characteristics likely to be associated with the behaviors at either end of the arrow. The arrowhead always denotes the presence of the listed attribute(s), whereas the tail end always denotes the absence of the same attribute(s).

tion of these arrows to the various crime behaviors displayed in the superimposed MDS diagram depict the nature of the relationship between the two sets of data, these being the patterns of crime behaviors and offender characteristics.

Core Principles Underpinning the CAP Models

This chapter has thus far provided a basic explanation of the statistical tool of MDS and how it is used to analyze and display patterns inherent to crime behaviors. This was followed by an explanation of the relationships between crime behaviors and offender characteristics and how these relationships are displayed by the use of large arrows (or lines, as in the case of serial arson discussed in Chapter 9). The integration of these two types of analysis, that is, the superimposition of the arrows on top of the MDS diagram, form the basis of a **CAP model**. The objective of the remainder of this chapter will be to explain in generic terms how these models can be systematically interpreted and thus used as a guide for the development of a criminal profile.

At the outset, a number of core principles concerning the structure and design of the CAP models need to be clearly understood. First, the CAP models in Chapters 7–9 each reflect totally separate studies concerning the crime behaviors and offender characteristics of serial rape (Chapter 7), sexual/serial murder (Chapter 8) and serial arson (Chapter 9). Consequently, these models are only applicable to their respective offense types. Accordingly, the CAP model depicted in Chapter 7 for serial rape should not be applied to or combined with, for example, any of the material in respect of serial arson contained in Chapter 9.

Second, regarding the general design of the three CAP models, it should be clearly understood that each model consists of four separate diagrams. The basis to all four diagrams in each of the CAP models is the MDS analysis of crime behaviors for the studied offense modality (i.e., sexual murder, serial rape, or serial arson). What differs across the four diagrams are the superimposed arrows (or lines in the case of the serial arson model) that depict the various offender characteristics and crime features, which have been linked to the patterns of crime behaviors depicted in the MDS diagram. Four separate diagrams are used simply for clarity in displaying the position of the arrows (or lines in Chapter 9) relative to the patterns of crime behaviors in the MDS diagram. The first diagram in each of the three CAP models always presents a depiction of the MDS analysis of crime behaviors without any arrows. The purpose of this first diagram in each of the models is to provide a clear depiction of the patterns inherent to the analyzed crime behaviors. The subsequent three diagrams in each CAP model present exactly the same MDS diagram with differing arrows at differing positions depicting related victim characteristics, offender characteristics, or interaction characteristics.* In principle, therefore, a CAP model could also be represented by a single MDS diagram that features all of the differing arrows (or lines) superimposed simultaneously on top of the one diagram. However, the clarity of such a diagram in discerning the proximity and therefore relationships between the differing variables would be compromised. Consequently, the use of the CAP models involves a cumulative process involving all four diagrams. That is, the prediction of offender characteristics based on observed crime behaviors is enhanced when the relationships inferred from all four of the diagrams are integrated and used in combination with each other. To use any less than all of the diagrams effectively equates to disregarding potential information concerning an offender that may have been derived from another diagram.

A final feature of the CAP models is their segmentation and appearance. All of the diagrams in the three CAP models displayed respectively in Chap-

---

* Some variation in these sets of data exist in the context of the CAP model for serial arson.

ters 7–9 typically feature a centrally located ellipse-shaped circle from which four lines extend to effectively segment the MDS diagram into four general regions. Additionally, within each of the MDS diagrams various small icons (typically represented by such shapes as circles, squares, crosses, etc.) are used. The significance of these variously shaped icons and segmentations in the diagrams are more relevant to the interpretation of the models with commonly occurring behavioral clusters and their relevance with previous research concerning offender typologies. Consequently, for the purpose of understanding the basic principles for interpreting a CAP model for operational use such borders and differently shaped icons can be overlooked. At this juncture it is more important to appreciate the relative positions of the icons (irrespective of their shape) relative to each other and the superimposed arrows within the MDS diagrams.

Basic Interpretation Principles

At its most fundamental level the concept of criminal profiling is a form of retro-classification *(2)*. Through the study of crime behaviors and related offender characteristics of past cases of sexual murder, for example, some insight can be gained about the perpetrator of a current case of sexual murder based on the similarities the current case may have with those studied previously. Because the CAP models are based on studies of samples of sexual murder, serial rape, and serial arson crimes, they provide a mechanism for identifying behavioral patterns apparent in each of these respective crime modalities. The process of constructing a criminal profile therefore principally involves identifying the behavioral variables evident in a crime under examination and then matching such variables with those identified in the appropriate CAP model. Although this may initially appear to be a somewhat mechanical procedure, some skill is required in discerning behavioral subtleties and gauging the probability of the related characteristics based on the particular circumstances of the case under consideration.

To understand the basic principles for using a CAP model to profile a sexual murder, refer to Fig. 6.3. The very first step will always involve a careful evaluation of the behaviors evident in the crime in question. The present hypothetical example will deal with the investigation of a murdered woman. The victim's clothing is observed to be torn/ripped and there is evidence of sexual assault. The autopsy indicates that the victim died as a result of stab wounds. It is also evident that one of the victim's nipples has been bitten off. Further forensic examination of the corpse indicates that the victim had been gagged and tortured. Because this crime is representative of a sexual murder,

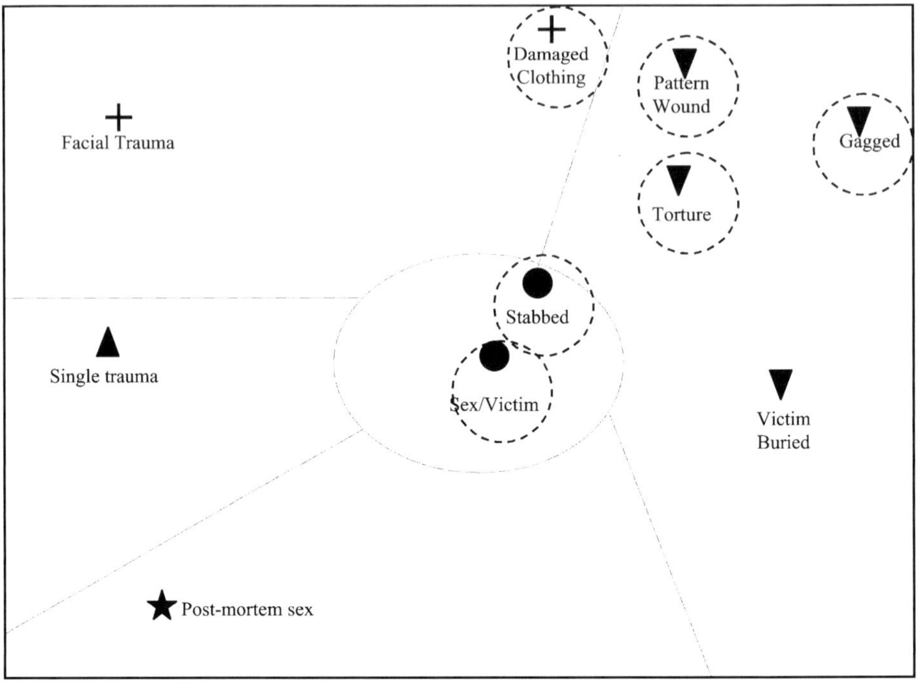

Fig. 6.3. Each of the behaviors evident in the crime being profiled are matched with corresponding icons from the multidimensional scaling diagram of the Crime Action Profiling model. Each of the relevant crime behaviors is circled.

the CAP model presented in Chapter 8 and specifically Figs. 8.1–8.4 would normally be used. However, in the present hypothetical example, the simplified diagrams contained in Fig. 6.3–6.8 will be relied on and referred to in this chapter. By referring to the first diagram (Fig. 6.3) in the CAP model, each of the behaviors just described would be matched and marked with the appropriate crime behavior icon in Fig. 6.3. Consequently, the corresponding crime behavior variables depicted in the MDS diagram of Fig. 6.3 are sex/victim, stabbed, damaged clothing, torture, gagged, and pattern wound.* Figure 6.3 illustrates the process whereby crime behavior icons in the MDS diagram are identified (i.e., encircled for ease of identification in this explanation) with those evident in the hypothetical crime.

All of the MDS diagrams in the three CAP models feature horizontal and vertical lines that bisect the MDS diagrams at a roughly central location.

*Biting off the victim's nipple is an example of a pattern wound.

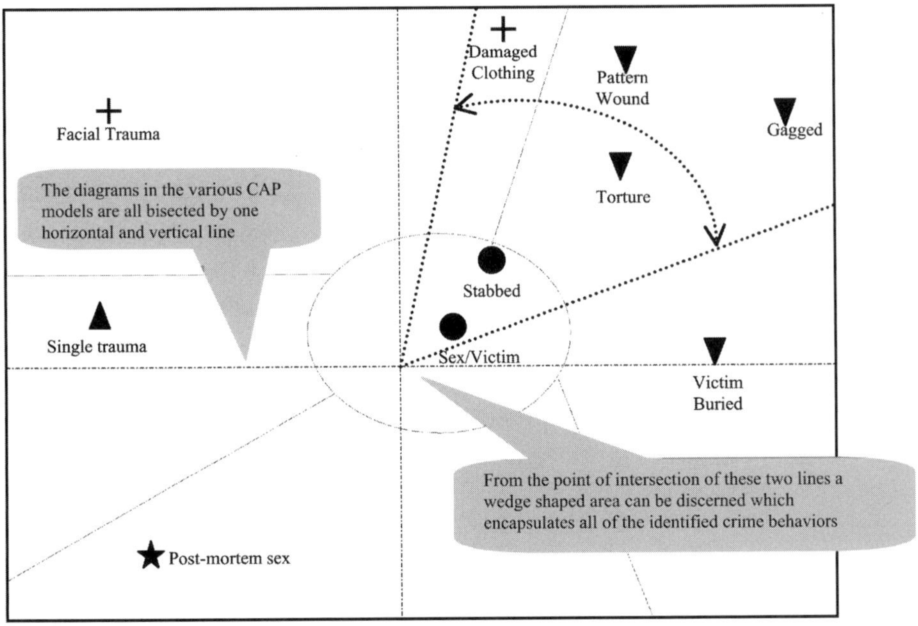

Fig. 6.4. A wedge-shaped region that encompasses all the relevant crime behavior icons should be identified from the point of intersection of the two bisecting lines found in each of the CAP models.

The intersection between these two lines is the central point of axis on which the position of all the arrows listing the offender characteristics are superimposed on the MDS diagrams.* From this central point of axis, a wedge-shaped area should be capable of identification within each of the MDS diagrams that encompasses the region containing all of the previously identified crime behavior icons. This process is displayed in Fig. 6.4. In undertaking this task, there are two important considerations. First, when identifying a wedge region in the MDS diagram it is important to ensure that the borders of this region encompass all of the previously identified crime behavior icons relevant to the crime under examination. The fact that other crime behavior icons not actually observed in the crime under examination may also be encompassed in this region is unimportant. Second, it should be understood that the point of intersection formed from the two axis lines do not necessarily bisect the MDS diagram at a perfectly central location. Nonetheless, it is the

*In the circumstance of the CAP model in Chapter 9, it is this same point of intersection from which all lines extend.

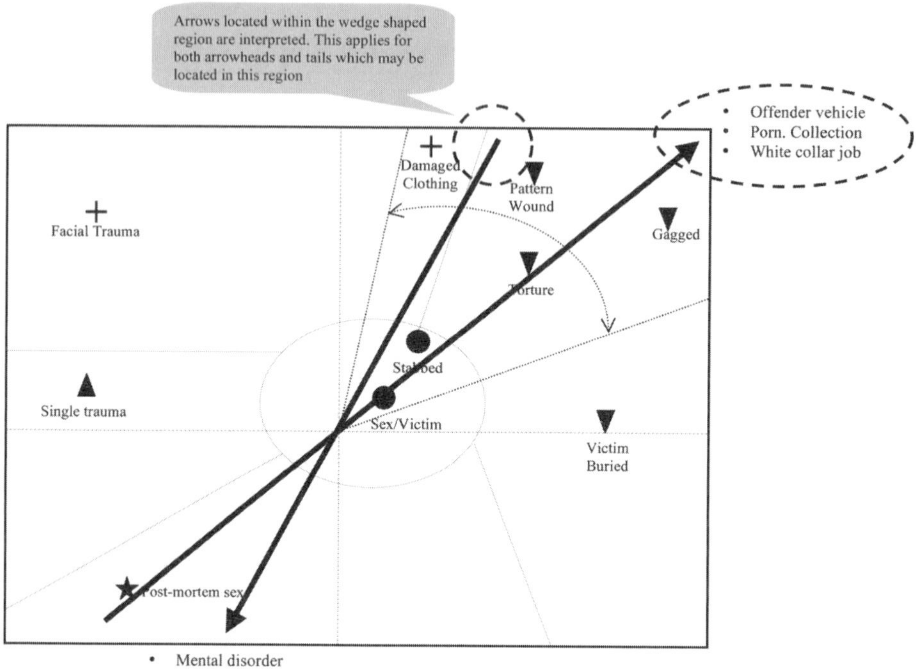

Fig. 6.5. The arrows located within the wedge-shaped region encompassing the identified crime behaviors can now be interpreted. These characteristics may be attributed to the probable offender(s). This process of interpretation is repeated for all three diagrams containing offender/crime characteristic arrows. All identified features cumulatively form the predictions of a criminal profile.

point of intersection identified by these two lines (and not some estimation of where the center of the diagram may be) that should always be used.

Having estimated an approximate wedge-shaped region in the MDS diagram, the process of predicting associated offender characteristics is a matter of referencing and interpreting the various arrows located within this same region in each of the MDS diagrams. There are two crucial issues to bear in mind when undertaking this task. First, it is vital to remember that characteristics derived through this process apply to both ends of any arrow (i.e., arrowheads as well as tails) that may come within the delineated wedge region.* Second, this procedure of identifying crime behaviors and then matching the associated offender characteristics is a collective process derived from all of the MDS diagrams displaying offender/crime characteristic arrows.

* In the circumstance of Chapter 9, an extension of the line in the opposite direction.

Figure 6.5 illustrates this procedure with the offender characteristics derived from a set of arrows that fall within the wedge region in only one hypothetical diagram. The arrowhead indicates that associated with the identified crime behaviors will be an offender who possesses a vehicle, a collection of pornographic materials, and who works in a white-collar job. The second arrow that falls within the wedge area has its tail in the region indicating that, in conjunction with the characteristics already predicted, the offender is unlikely to be suffering from a mental disorder. As indicated previously, this process of identifying offender characteristics would be repeated on the two other MDS diagrams of the same CAP model. The collection of all characteristics derived through this process on all diagrams then forms the basis of the predictions comprising a criminal profile. It should perhaps be remembered that the predictions made are just that—they are not certainties and are informed by probability (i.e., the likelihood of any given factor being present or absent).

Advanced Principles

It needs to be emphasized that the material canvassed thus far throughout this chapter is specifically designed to facilitate a fundamental understanding of the principles for interpreting CAP models when seeking to formulate a criminal profile. It is therefore important to thoroughly understand these basic procedures, as the advanced principles articulated herein essentially represent more sophisticated elaborations of these basic principles.

Interpreting the Arrows as Sliding Scales

Thus far, the principles for interpreting the offender and crime characteristics listed beside the various arrows have been explained in terms of being either present or absent, dependent on the position of the arrowhead or tail. This procedure represents a simplified way of understanding the functional properties behind these arrows. However, their interpretation is better conceptualized as two opposing polarities along a continuum. Consequently, the arrowhead, or positive polarity, of an arrow represents a high or affirmative probability for the listed characteristics, whereas the tail, or negative polarity, of an arrow represents a low probability for the same characteristic(s). By this conceptualization of the arrows as continuums, the strength and nature of the relationships between the characteristics listed beside each arrow and the individual crime behaviors in the MDS diagrams can be better interpreted. Figure 6.6 provides an illustration of this concept. Based on their proximity near the arrowhead there is a very strong relationship between the victim being buried and the listed characteristics. A weaker, but nonetheless, still present

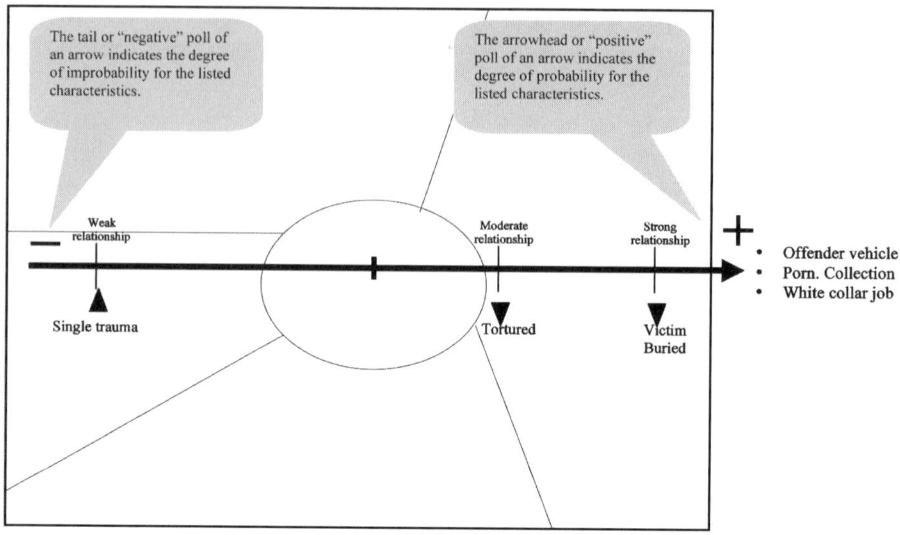

Fig. 6.6. The interpretation of the offender/crime characteristics listed near each arrow should be interpreted in terms of a weighted scale rather than in a categorical sense of presence or absence. The position of a crime behavior along the length of an arrow indicates broadly the probability or improbability of the characteristic(s).

relationship exists between the same offender characteristics and the crime behavior icon of the victim being tortured. Conversely, there is an extremely weak, or more likely, no relationship between the listed offender characteristics for the arrow and the crime behavior of a single point of trauma on the victim. These factors in interpreting the CAP models can be more precisely gauged and expressed in a written criminal profile wherein emphasis can be placed on the relative strengths of these relationships (i.e., probability of being observed in the offender).

Another important aspect surrounding the interpretation of the arrows relates to some of the characteristics assigned to the arrows. For ease of explanation, the characteristics referred to thus far have dealt with variables that can be easily defined as either present or absent, such as, for example, whether or not the offender possesses a vehicle. Some of the offender characteristics listed adjacent to the arrows are not amenable to such interpretation. One example of this is an offender's likely age. Consequently, the significance of these variables necessitates their interpretation along a weighted scale. Thus, using the example of an offender's possible age, the positive arrowhead denotes an offender who is likely to be older, whereas the negative tail of the arrow denotes an offender who is likely to be younger.

Regional Interpretation of Crime Behaviors

Another nuance to the interpretation of the CAP models relates to the identification of relevant crime behavior icons and the concomitant arrows. The basic procedure articulated thus far involves identifying the two outlying behaviors to form borders from which a conceptual wedge can be identified within the MDS diagram. All arrows within this designated wedge region can then be used for the prediction of characteristics. Although this is a method by which the CAP models can be interpreted, it does resort, in part, to a somewhat categorical process, using affixed borders to form the conceptual wedge region in the MDS diagrams. A more sophisticated method for interpretation involves assessing the proximity of each of the relevant crime behavior icons with any neighboring arrows. In many circumstances, this technique will result in a similar interpretation of the CAP models akin to the basic procedure because of the overall structure of the crime behavior icons displayed in the MDS diagrams. The advantage of this method of interpretation, however, comes from the consideration of arrows that typically fall outside the conceptual wedge region but nonetheless share a close proximity with one of the crime behavior icons. An example of this is when a crime behavior delineates the border of the wedge region.

Figure 6.7 provides an illustration of this concept. The left border of the wedge region generated by following the basic procedure in this example is created by the crime behavior of damaged clothing. Although two arrows fall to the right of this crime behavior icon and are within the conceptualized wedge region, a third arrow to the left also shares a close proximity with this damaged clothing icon. In following the basic approach of interpreting the CAP models, this third arrow would not normally be considered. Gauging the individual proximity of the crime behaviors with any neighboring arrows, however, indicates some relationship between this variable and the arrow.

Commonality in Crime Behaviors

One final nuance to the interpretation of the CAP models involves specific consideration of the overall positions the crime behavior icons occupy in the MDS diagrams. As explained in the initial section of this chapter, the MDS diagrams represent an analysis of crime behaviors in each of the respective crime modalities. The purpose of this analysis is to identify the relationships between these variables illustrated by their proximity to one another.

One of the reasons why MDS was used in developing the CAP models was to offer some explanation concerning the commonalties inherent to the various crime behaviors. This concept will be discussed in far more detail in subsequent chapters dealing with the theoretical considerations underpinning

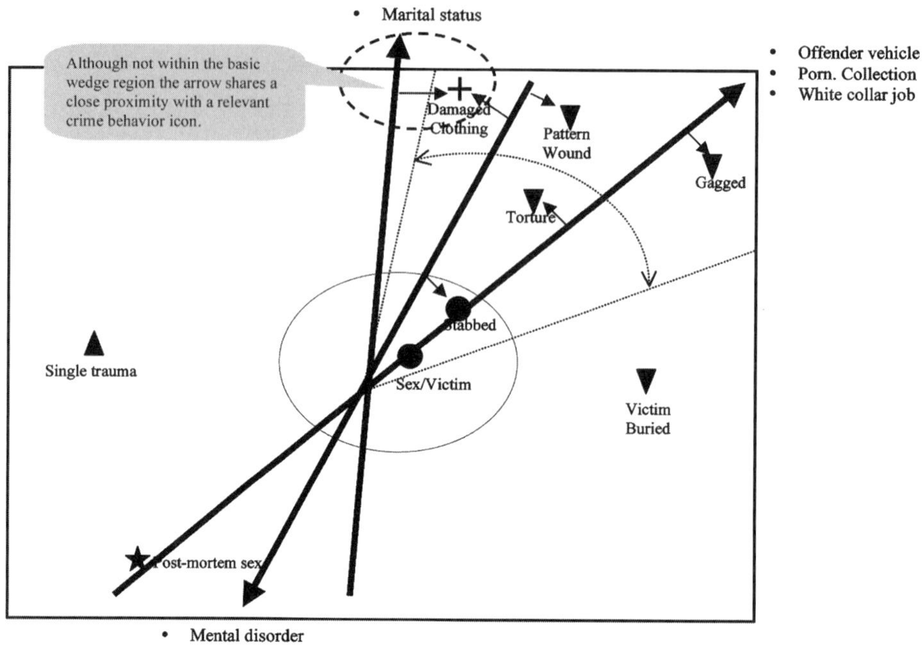

Fig. 6.7. A more refined method of interpreting the relationship between the variables in a CAP model involves examining the proximity of each of the individual crime scene behaviors in relation to the arrows.

the models. However, in the context of the present chapter, it is important to appreciate that the priority of these crime behaviors for the purpose of developing a profile varies depending on their relative position in the MDS diagram. The closer crime behavior icons appear to the center of a MDS diagram, the more common they are in comparison to those positioned in the outlying areas of the diagram.* However, this does not mean that some crime behaviors are invalid to some degree, but instead indicates that some behaviors are likely to be commonly occurring and characteristic of a particular type of crime in general rather than being a distinctive aspect of behavior particular to the offense under investigation. A hypothetical example may be the presence of

*All of the CAP models feature an elipse in the center of the diagram. This elipse can be used as a rudimentary guide to judge the significance of the crime behaviors under consideration. Those crime behaviors located within the elipse have been found to be quite common and thus nondiscriminatory to the particular crime modality.

stab wounds on a victim in a sexual murder. The location of this variable in the center of a MDS diagram indicates that the stabbing of a victim is a common feature observed in sexual murder offenses.

The positions of the arrows are aligned to these same concepts concerning the priority of their corresponding variables. Crime behavior icons that are located closer to the center of a MDS diagram also hold a roughly central position with any of the arrows. In line with the previous explanation of a weighted interpretation of the arrows, such intermediary positions along their planes indicate a weak or ambivalent relationship between the crime behaviors and the characteristics listed beside the arrow.

How these principles can inform the development of a criminal profile is in discerning the strength and value of the relationships indicated by the positions of the crime behavior icons relative to any of the arrows. Essentially, a descending order of emphasis can be adopted when interpreting the relationships. That is, stronger and more prominent relationships (and therefore predictions) can be made based on icons found in the outlying regions of the MDS diagram (relative to the arrows), whereas weaker (i.e., less prominent) predictions arise from variables found closer to the center of the MDS diagram. Figure 6.8 provides a simplified illustration of these concepts. The encircled crime behavior icon of the victim having been sexually assaulted (i.e., sex/victim) is located in a roughly central position on the MDS diagram. This central position indicates that this behavior is actually very common to sexual murder crimes. Although this behavior has been observed in the case being considered, its occurrence is not a particularly discriminatory feature of the offender being profiled. Consistent with this is the location of the sex/victim icon that appears roughly midway along the arrow, indicating a weak or ambivalent relationship between this crime behavior and the corresponding listed offender characteristics. Consequently, any interpretation derived from the observation of this behavior should be given a low degree of emphasis. In contrast, however, the crime behavior of pattern wound appears in an outlying region towards the top right of the MDS diagram. Consequently, the position of this behavior is far more likely to be a discriminatory feature of the particular offender being profiled. Similarly, the position of this icon relative to the arrow suggests the presence of a prominent positive relationship between this crime behavior and the corresponding listed offender characteristics. Accordingly, when constructing a criminal profile, predictions based on the relationship between these variables should be given greater emphasis over that derived from the sex/victim icon.

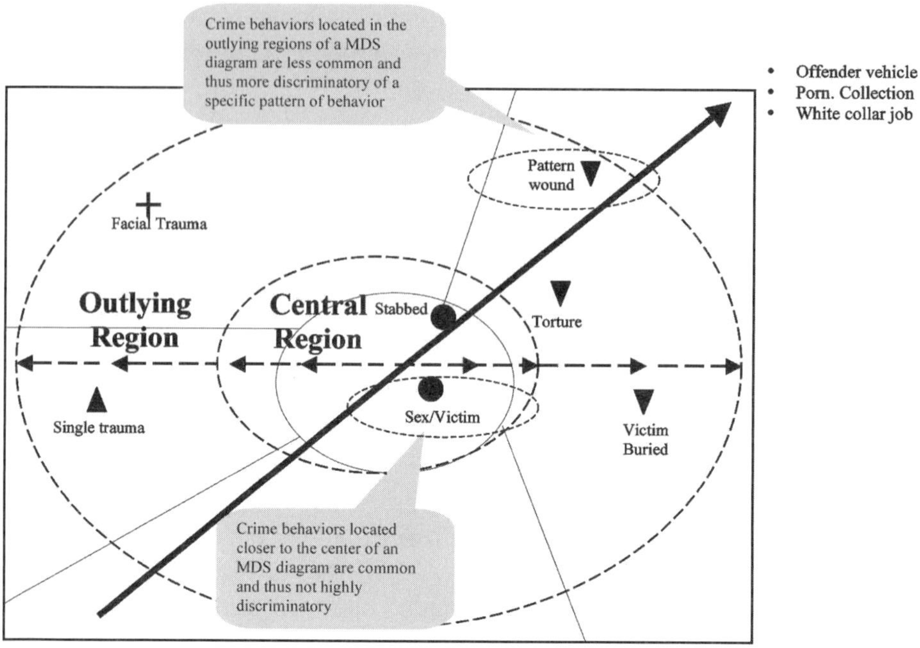

Fig. 6.8. The center of a multidimensional scaling diagram serves as a point of locus from which the positions of all variables relative to each other are calculated. Radiating outward from the center of the diagram the position of the variables denotes their commonality. Consequently, crime behaviors positioned closer to the center of the diagram are common, whereas those positioned further away in the outlying region are more distinctive.

Conclusion

This chapter articulated a basic, generic method for the interpretation and use of the various CAP models. The initial section offered a rudimentary explanation of some of the statistical procedures inherent to the development of these models. The focus of this exposition, however, was not to explain the research and statistical methodologies employed in the development of the models, but rather to explain their functioning. By focusing on these concepts it is hoped that a user-friendly understanding of the models can be achieved to guide in the evaluation of a given crime for the purpose of developing a criminal profile.

It should be apparent that the research and procedures of CAP are quite different from other approaches to criminal profiling in that CAP offers structured models that serve as **mechanisms** for the profiling of violent crimes.

This differs significantly from other approaches that espouse a range of offender taxonomies and/or maxims that require a considerable amount of subjective interpretation in their application for the development of a criminal profile. One example is the organized and disorganized offender typology *(3)*. This typology consists of two mutually exclusive templates (i.e., a dichotomy) for sexual murderers that are differentiated by the degree of behavioral sophistication argued to be discernable from crimes of these offenders. Thus, organized offenders are characterized by a high degree of planning in their offenses, whereas disorganized offenders are characterized by a low level of planning. It is argued by proponents of this dichotomy that its application to profiling can be accomplished by matching the behavioral features evident in the crime under consideration with either of the two categories.

Unfortunately, however, identifying which behaviors exhibited in the crime under consideration belong to which of the two mutually exclusive categories is often problematic because combinations of crime behaviors indicative of both categories invariably arise. That is, behaviors indicative of both an organized and disorganized offender are frequently observed in the same crime. Consequently, the practical application of this dichotomy often involves the highly subjective assessment of identifying which behaviors from each category are appropriate for the development of a profile. It appears that the problems encountered in the application of this categorical distinction in part prompted the invention of the mixed offender category *(4)* subsequent to the development of the original dichotomy. However, in the author's view, the mixed offender category only serves to highlight the problem inherent to any type of classification used for profiling that is heavily reliant on the use of categorical constructs. Unfortunately, crime behaviors rarely fit neatly and conveniently into discrete categories.

In contrast to the organized–disorganized dichotomy, the interpretive procedures of the CAP models discussed in this chapter are not category-dependent. Segments are instead formed by the crime behaviors present in any given case using the model. Wherever the behaviors are located in the model determines the segment, which in turn determines the relevance or otherwise of observed offender characteristics. In this way, constructing a criminal profile using a CAP model does not involve any rigid template concerning a typical offender or his or her crime scene behaviors. Instead, the CAP models serve as a responsive mechanism by which virtually any combination of behaviors evident in a particular crime can be specifically and systematically assessed. Thus, predictions concerning an offender's characteristics are generated in direct response to the particular combination of behaviors observed in the crime and matched with the variables contained in the appropriate model. In this way, the determination of associations between behaviors and related characteristics is not a wholly subjective process. Most importantly, the CAP method can be followed and readily replicated by others.

In conclusion, it should be emphasized that the CAP models presented in this book provide a mechanism for the identification of links between discernable patterns in crime behaviors and offender characteristics typically associated with those crime behaviors. The interpretation of information derived from the CAP models, which is used as a guide for the developing of a criminal profile, should always involve a considered evaluation of the specific facts and circumstances surrounding the crime under review. In so doing, it should always be remembered that the exercise is one involving probability rather than certainty, and one should bear this in mind when attempting to interpret and assess the importance of any given variable for the purpose of developing a criminal profile.

References

1. Coxon, A.P.M. (1982). The user's guide to multidimensional scaling. London: Heinemann.
2. Turco, R.N. (1990). Psychological profiling. International Journal of Offender Therapy and Comparative Criminology, 34, 147–154.
3. Ressler, R.K., Burgess, A., Douglas, J.E. (1988). Sexual homicide: Patterns and motives. New York: Lexington Books.
4. Kocsis, R.N., Irwin, H.J., Hayes, A.F. (1998). Organized and disorganized behaviour syndromes in arsonists: A validation study of a psychological profiling concept. Psychiatry, Psychology & Law, 5, 117–130.

Chapter 7

Criminal Profiling of Serial Rape Offenses

Summary

This chapter reports on the findings of an original empirical study into serial rape profiling. The statistical procedure of multidimensional scaling was employed to produce a five-cluster model of serial rapist behavior. First, a central cluster was identified that represented behaviors common to all patterns of serial rape. Second, four distinct outlying patterns were identified as demonstrating distinct offense styles, these being assigned the descriptive labels of brutality, intercourse, chaotic, and ritual. Further analysis also identified a range of offender characteristics that are associated with each of these crime behavior patterns.

Key Words: Criminal profiling; serial rape offenses.

Introduction

It appears that in the study of serial violent crimes for the specific purpose of criminal profiling, a very limited number of original, quantitative, peer-reviewed studies have been published *(1)*. Instead, scholarly activity in this area has been dominated by articles oriented more toward conceptual discussion of issues related to criminal profiling *(2–13)*. Therefore, the objective of the study canvassed in this chapter was to undertake an original, empirically based analysis of serial rape behavior patterns and explore their respective association with offender characteristics. Within this context there are three main bodies of research relevant to the criminal profiling of serial rape offenses. These are the studies by Groth et al. *(14)*, the work of the FBI's Behavioral Science Unit *(15,16)*, and the research of Canter and Heritage *(17)*. Each of these bodies of research is discussed herein.

From: *Criminal Profiling: Principles and Practice*
By: R. N. Kocsis © Humana Press Inc., Totowa, NJ

One of the earliest studies relevant to rape profiling was undertaken by Groth et al. *(14)*. These authors proposed a typology of rape offenders based on the tenet that rape is a pseudosexual act in which sex merely serves as a vehicle for the primary motivations of power and aggression. In this typology, Groth et al. *(14)* identified three broad patterns of rape. First is the anger rapist who uses more force than necessary for compliance in the assault and engages in a variety of sexual acts that are degrading to the victim. These sexual assaults are characterized by considerable physical violence and brutality and are said to represent a conscious act of anger and rage towards the victim. Second is the power rapist who seeks to establish power and control over the victim, to assert his potency, mastery, and identity. Consequently, the amount of force and threat used depends on the degree of submission by the victim. Third and finally is the sadistic rapist who exhibits a combination of both sexual and aggressive components. Aggression is eroticized and the offender is typically aroused and excited by the victim's maltreatment, torment, and suffering. These assaults often involve bondage, torture, and considerable abuse and injury to the victim. Although a number of further psychiatric typologies have arisen *(18)* subsequent to the work of Groth et al. *(14)*, they are essentially elaborations on the original concepts espoused by Groth et al. *(14)*.

The second body of research relevant to the present study originates from the FBI's Behavioral Science Unit. Arguably one of the most cited studies in the area of criminal profiling was undertaken by this group in the 1980s and involved the analysis of 36 incarcerated sexual murderers. The result of this study was the invention of the organized–disorganized behavior dichotomy. The underlying premise informing this dichotomy is the interpretation of crimes by their level of behavioral sophistication and corresponding offender characteristics. Thus, the organized category represents a methodical, premeditated crime with corresponding offender characteristics, such as maturity, resourcefulness, and typically, sexual perversion. The disorganized category, however, represents a haphazard, almost random crime with the corresponding inverse offender characteristics of immaturity, opportunism, and a likelihood of some mental disorder *(15)*.

Despite the renown of this research, empirical replication of this dichotomy has been disappointingly lacking. One of the few replications, such as that undertaken by Kocsis et al. *(19)*, found that although the basic concept of interpreting crimes by their level of behavioral sophistication holds some merit, a more robust mechanism for the interpretation of crime behaviors is required beyond a simplistic dichotomy. An example of a limitation to this dichotomy is its failure to make any distinction between commonly occurring behaviors and those that are discriminate of (i.e., unique to) a particular offender. As mentioned in Chapter 6, if an offender inflicts stab wounds in the commission of a sexual murder, this may not actually be a unique behavioral clue about a particular offender, but rather, a very common behavior observed in most sexual murder offenses. Thus, the categorical distinctions of the organized–disorganized dichotomy may lead to the prediction of some erroneous feature based on the observation of stab wounds when, in fact, it may simply represent a behavioral attribute common to sexual murders in general. Indeed, this failing to empirically distinguish between common behaviors and those that are discriminatory of a specific individual is a failing that appears to prevail throughout much of the literature on criminal profiling in general.

In recognition of the popularity of their research into sexual murderers, and guided by the typologies originally devised by Groth et al. *(14)*, the FBI Behavioral Science Unit undertook research in the area of recidivistic sexual assault. The outcome of this research was the compilation of demographic data pertinent to serial rape offenders *(16)*. Regrettably, a weakness of this research is its failure to describe how this material may be coherently integrated with the organized–disorganized dichotomy, the categories described by Groth et al. *(14)*, and the data interpreted to systematically construct a criminal profile.

The third relevant contribution to rape profiling was the study undertaken by Canter and Heritage *(17)*. These authors argue that the development of empirically valid criminal profiling techniques requires the study of offender behaviors as distinct from their inferred motives. Canter and Heritage *(17)* relied on a basic hypothesis of criminal profiling that offenders differ in their behaviors when perpetrating a crime and it is these differences in behavior that relate to their characteristics. Consequently, any attempt to understand the behaviors that occur in an offense requires the classification of offense behaviors as distinct from the classification of the offender in psychological or social terms *(17)*. In effect, behavior variations in sexual attacks indicate the different modes of relationship offenders share with their victims. Consequently, previous offender typologies, such as those espoused by Groth et al. *(14)*, that combine inferred motivations with behaviors are argued to be empirically flawed *(17)*.

Following these principles, Canter and Heritage *(17)* studied a sample of rape cases. The results of their study yielded two interesting findings. First, it concluded that the central theme underlying the commission of rape offenses was the treatment of the victim as an impersonal object. This conclusion was similar to that drawn previously by Scully and Marolla *(20)* who proposed that the motivations for rape primarily involve impersonal drives associated with criminality. This conception of rapist behavior is contrary to that of Groth et al. *(14)* who, as previously mentioned, argue that the underlying theme to rape is the sexual expression of anger and power.

The second important finding to emerge from Canter and Heritage's *(17)* study was the identification of five distinct behavioral patterns in the commission of rape offenses. Canter and Heritage *(17)* labeled the first pattern the intimacy pattern, represented by behaviors indicative of the offender attempting to establish intimacy with the victim. Canter and Heritage *(17)* argued that this pattern was in keeping with the views of Marshall *(21)* who proposed that rape represented a means for an offender to compensate for an inability to establish normal relations with a partner. The second pattern was labeled sexuality and features intercourse with the victim as a crucial element of the assault. A third pattern, labeled violence, was used to explain an inherent theme of violence against the victim and thus concurs partially with the theories of Groth et al. *(14)*. The fourth pattern, labeled impersonal, is comprised of behaviors indicative of a purely impersonal treatment of the victim. The fifth pattern, labeled criminality, sought to describe behaviors associated with criminal actions that were not overtly sexual in purpose.

Although suggesting an empirical approach to the identification of patterns in rapist offense behaviors, Canter and Heritage's *(17)* study fails to address the issue of associating these crime behavior patterns with offender characteristics. Although their study reveals a valuable method for the interpretation of crime behavior patterns, it does not provide information on the practical application of their research to sexual assault profiling.

In summary, therefore, the primary objective of the study discussed in this chapter was to analyze serial rape crime behaviors as distinct from inferred motivations while also using some form of direct statistical analysis to match offender characteristics with the identified patterns in crime behavior. An inherent component of this study involved using a method of analysis for the identification of common behaviors from those that are representative of discriminatory patterns.

Additionally, the present study employed the selection criteria for serial rape offenses previously discussed in Chapter 5. The central thesis informing these criteria was the identification of offenders based on behavioral characteristics indicative of an individual's psychological make-up to commit further serial, sexually violent offenses. The criteria discussed in Chapter 5 serve to establish some uniformity in the classification of serial crime and arguably reduce the potentially confounding surplus of cases included in the analysis. For example, these criteria would exclude cases in which there was a prior relationship between the victim and offender and the offender had sexually assaulted the same victim at various times. An illustration of such a circumstance is domestic sexual assault between spouses. In the past, the lack of uniform definition for serial offenders has led to substantially divergent sampling procedures in previous serial murderer studies with corresponding variations in research outcomes *(22–24)*.

It was hypothesized from the outset that the present study would have two outcomes. First, it would develop an empirical model for profiling serial rape offenses. This model would yield distinct behavioral patterns that could be empirically matched with discriminate offender characteristics. Second, the analysis of crime actions would also identify behaviors that were nondiscriminatory and thus commonly observable in all serial rape behavior patterns.

*Methods**

Datapool and Data Screening Process

The data used in this study consisted of 62 sexual assault cases from 1960 to 1998. All offenders in the sample had been convicted of at least one sexual assault. In some circumstances, cases had missing details concerning some variables. To achieve a stable and internally consistent refined data pool for subsequent analysis, variables were screened and marked for retention in the data pool if they demonstrated sufficient non-missing entries and sufficient variability across categories for each variable. The screening process involved computing frequency distributions for all variables in the data pool. Variables presenting predominantly constant data values were removed before analysis, as were variables that were missing for more than 50% of the cases in the data pool. This preliminary screening process retained a sizeable number of variables that required further condensation before analysis.

Condensation of the Variables

To facilitate data analysis and interpretation, conceptually similar categories for each variable were collapsed with a view to producing dichotomous (0, 1) measures having a reasonable number of category 1 responses. Most variables were recoded on a presence–absence basis, whereas others were recoded into less–more-type categories. Some variables having multiple categories were dummy coded into several dichotomous variables (e.g., the variables for initial contact location, crime scene location, type of weapon used,

*Readers are reminded that the material provided here is to offer a more theoretically oriented understanding of how the CAP models were originally constructed. However, as explained in Chapter 6, an understanding of this material is not essential for the pragmatic construction of a criminal profile where the procedures discussed in Chapter 6 can simply be used.

etc.). Variables with very few or no category 1 responses were deleted from the data pool.

As a result of this data screening and variable condensation process, more than 200 variables were reduced to a final set of 115 variables. Variables were broadly grouped into conceptual sets for subsequent analyses: victim characteristics (6 variables), offender characteristics (33 variables), offender–victim interaction characteristics (23 variables), and crime scene characteristics (53 variables). All variable labels and extended names used for the multidimensional scaling (MDS) diagrams are shown in Appendix B.

Analytical Process

The analysis proceeded through several discrete stages. The first stage employed a non-metric MDS analysis of the 53 dichotomous crime scene characteristics to identify the appropriate number of dimensions from the range of two- to five-dimensional solutions for interpretation *(25)*. This analysis was accomplished using the MDS program in SYSTAT 9.0. The scaling process was controlled using the Guttman coefficient of alienation minimization criterion and the Jaccard measure of binary similarity. The two-dimensional MDS solution that emerged from this stage was retained for further analysis and interpretation.

The second stage of the process subjected the resulting MDS coordinates to cluster analysis to facilitate a regional interpretation of the dimensional solution *(26,27)*. Ward's minimum variance hierarchical cluster analysis was employed for this stage using the squared Euclidean distance measure of dissimilarity. The dimensional coordinates of the MDS solution were standardized (converted to *z*-scores) then plotted on to a scatterplot using cluster identifiers to differentiate the plotting symbols.

The third stage in the process focused on fitting external property vectors, using variables from the victim, offender, and offender–victim interaction variable sets, to the MDS coordinates for each of the 53 crime scene characteristics. A new data pool was constructed containing the standardized dimensional coordinates from the MDS analysis and conditional probabilities for each characteristic variable not employed in the first-stage MDS analysis (referred to as external variables). Each entry in the data pool for a combination of a specific external variable and crime scene characteristic was computed as the mean for that external variable within the category coded 1 for that specific crime scene characteristic. This mean was thus interpretable as the conditional probability that the variable (e.g., VSEX) equaled 1 (female) when a specific crime scene characteristic (e.g., BLNDFLDV) also equaled 1 (victim was blindfolded). These conditional probabilities became the external characteristic property vector variables, which were fitted to the MDS coordinates to aid in interpretation. Two additional statistical control variables were computed: one indicating the number of non-missing cases (out of 62 cases) for each crime scene variable and the other indicating the number of observations comprising the category coded as 1 for each crime scene characteristic.

Property fitting was accomplished using an extension of the multiple regression procedure for fitting direction cosines described by Kruskal and Wish (*26*, pp. 87–88). Each of the conditional probability variables within a specific conceptual set (e.g., victim characteristic set) were predicted from the standardized MDS coordinates using the set correlation analysis procedure in SYSTAT 9.0 (*see* Cohen and Cohen *[28]* for a discussion of set correlation as a multivariate relational technique). Both the predictor set (MDS coordinates), and criterion set (conditional probability variables), were partialed for the influence of the number of non-missing observations and observations comprising the category coded as 1, to control for the possible influences of missing data and small category 1 membership. The appropriate multivariate canonical correlation, associated with each variable set comprising the cluster for each vector was recorded and tested for overall significance. This process was repeated for the remaining conceptual sets (i.e., offender characteristics and offender–victim interaction characteristics).

Working at the univariate level, each significant external characteristic variable within a set was identified. The significance decision was based on the omnibus F-test for the regression analysis of that variable. Then, the standardized regression coefficients for each of the MDS dimensions for each significant variable within the set of interest were then cluster analyzed using Ward's method and Euclidean distance to identify the most appropriate number of clusters of characteristics. This was done to reduce empirically the number of distinct property vectors that would have to be fit, thus facilitating simpler and more straightforward interpretations. For each identified cluster of external characteristics, the standardized regression weights for each dimension were averaged across the variables comprising the cluster.* On separate MDS dimensional plots (one for each conceptual set of external vari-

---

*To illustrate the first few steps of the property fitting process, consider the steps taken to analyze the variables in the victim characteristics set. The six variables comprising this set were individually regressed onto the two standardized MDS dimension coordinates and the resulting standardized (β) weights for the two dimensions was recorded (thus, six distinct regression were run for this set, although the set correlation method in SYSTAT ran them all simultaneously). Out of the six original variables in the set, only the victim's marital status (VMARITAL) was not significantly predicted by the MDS coordinates and was therefore dropped from further consideration. The remaining set of weights (five variables by two weights) was

ables analyzed), the property vectors for each cluster of variables were fitted using the averaged regression β weights transformed to yield a specific vector angle that was then drawn onto the graph using an arrowhead. The angle computed ranged between 0 and 360° and thus directly indicated the direction that the association arrowhead should point.*

RESULTS

Multidimensional Scaling

Following the close examination of the two- through five-dimensional solutions, the two-dimensional solution was selected as most appropriate for interpretation (coefficient of alienation = 0.228; $R^2 = 0.795$). The higher-order dimensional solutions, although producing marginally better data fit, were conceptually more difficult to clearly interpret. Interpretability was the ultimate criterion to be met by the solution adopted and two dimensions proved most interpretable. Figure 7.1 shows the plot of the standardized coordinates for the two-dimensional MDS solution for the 53 crime scene characteristics.

The two-dimensional MDS coordinates were hierarchically clustered and five clusters of crime scene characteristics were identified. These clusters divided the two-dimensional space of crime scene characteristics into five non-overlapping regions. The five clusters of coordinates are marked by distinct plotting symbols in Fig. 7.1, in which the cluster regions have also been sketched in. Figure 7.1 could be interpreted in several ways, but one of the clearest ways is a regional interpretation. Crime scene characteristics appear-

---

(*continued from previous page*) cluster analyzed and three distinct clusters of variables were identified. One such cluster comprised the victim's sex (VSEX) and victim's age (VAGE) variables and the standardized weights for each dimension were averaged across the two giving an average β weight for dimension 1 and an average β weight for dimension 2. These two averaged weights then formed the basis for fitting the property vector to the two-dimensional MDS solution plot in Fig. 7.1.

*The specific formulas used for this transformation were as follows where *a* and *b* reflect the two dimensions that anchor the graph in question:

$$if(\beta_a > 0 \text{ and } \beta_b > 0\text{) angle} = \deg\left[(\cos^{-1}\beta_a / \sqrt{\beta_a^2 + \beta_b^2})\right]$$

$$if(\beta_a > 0 \text{ and } \beta_b < 0\text{) angle} = 360 - \deg\left[(\cos^{-1}\beta_a / \sqrt{\beta_a^2 + \beta_b^2})\right]$$

$$if(\beta_a < 0 \text{ and } \beta_b > 0\text{) angle} = 180 - \deg\left[(\cos^{-1}|\beta_a| / \sqrt{\beta_a^2 + \beta_b^2})\right]$$

$$if(\beta_a < 0 \text{ and } \beta_b < 0\text{) angle} = 180 + \deg\left[(\cos^{-1}|\beta_a| / \sqrt{\beta_a^2 + \beta_b^2})\right]$$

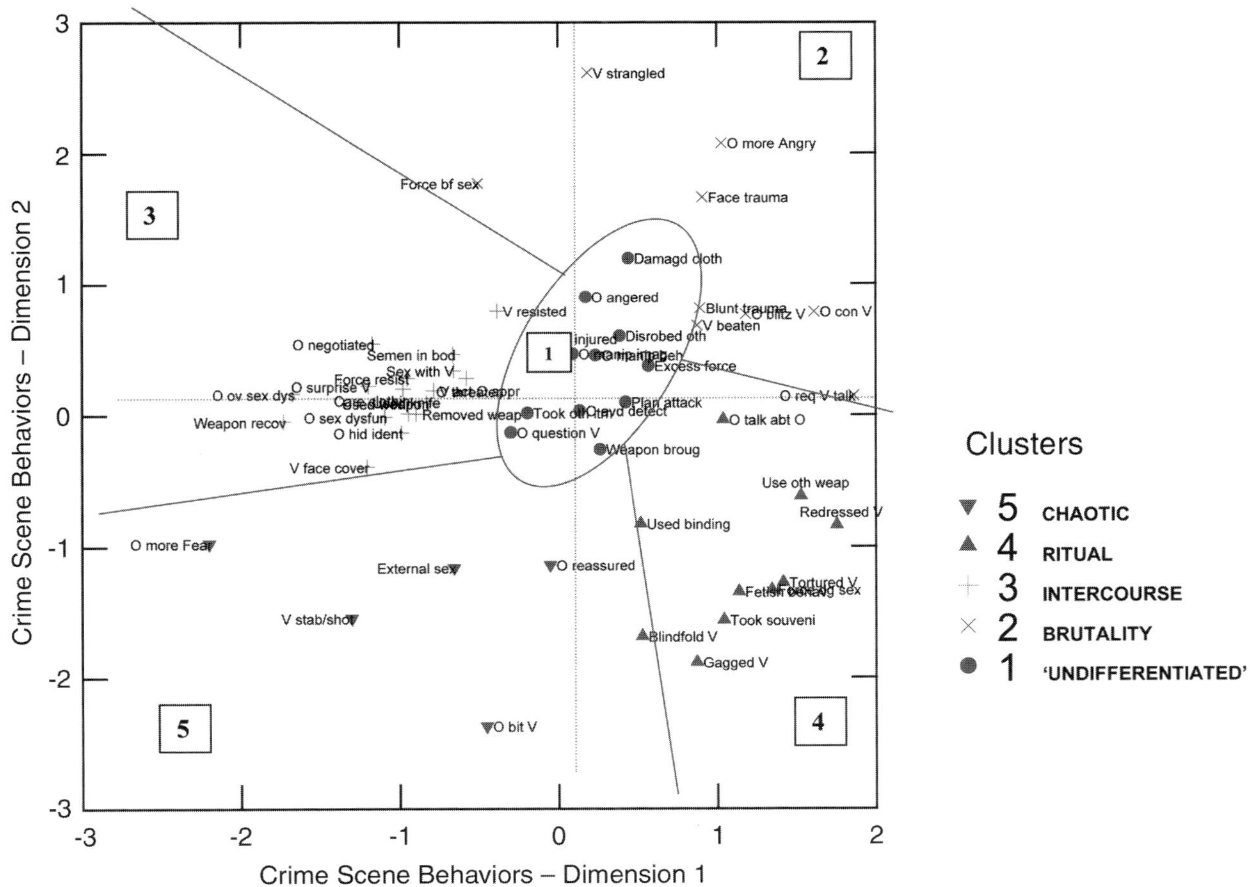

Fig. 7.1. Two-dimensional sexual assault crime scene behavior multidimensional scaling solution with coordinate cluster structure superimposed.

ing in the same region of the plot were inspected for common themes to aid in the interpretation of what each region might be indicating. The central cluster 1, surrounded by the ellipse, represented crime scene characteristics that were not clearly discriminated by the two-dimensional MDS structure—they were associated by virtue of having similar coordinate patterns centered on or near zero for each dimension. Thus, these particular crime scene characteristics were not very useful for distinguishing between different crime scenes with a view to inferring anything uniquely meaningful about crime scenes, hence the label undifferentiated. The four regions surrounding the central regions represented clusters of crime scene characteristics that tended to appear together sufficiently often to constitute a distinctive pattern.

Cluster 4, to the lower right of the central ellipse was labeled the *ritual* pattern because it seemed to capture a pattern of very violent crime scene characteristics, suggesting an element of deliberateness and calculation in the behaviors. Total dominance of the victim appears to be an underlying theme. Cluster 3, to the immediate left of the central ellipse was labeled the *intercourse* pattern because it seemed to capture crime scene characteristics suggestive of less violent intent in which the offender obviously intended to sexually assault the victim, frequently in an anonymous manner, and which involved either the offender hiding their identity or concealing the victim's face.

Cluster 2 was labeled *brutality* because it suggested a pattern of crime scene behaviors that had a very violent and forceful nature—an anger theme seemed to underscore this region. Supporting this interpretation is the very near proximity of crime scene characteristics from the undifferentiated cluster (e.g., damaging the victim's clothing [damaged cloth], offender being initially angered [O angered], and offender's use of excessive force [excess force]).

Finally, cluster 5 was labeled the *chaotic* pattern because the crime scene behaviors were suggestive of some mental instability being associated with the sexual assault. An interesting feature of this cluster is the nature of the characteristics that comprise it, namely the range of characteristic behaviors exhibited by the offender typically suggest contrition on the part of the offender. Supporting this idea is the very near proximity of crime scene characteristics from neighboring clusters (e.g., covering the victim's face [V face cover], offender hiding his own identity [O hid ident]), and blindfolding the victim [blindfold V]). Yet, certain violent acts (stabbing–shooting and biting) are also associated with this cluster.

External Property Vector Fitting

Figures 7.2 through 7.4 summarize the property vector fitting analyses designed to explicitly employ clusters of characteristics of the victim, the

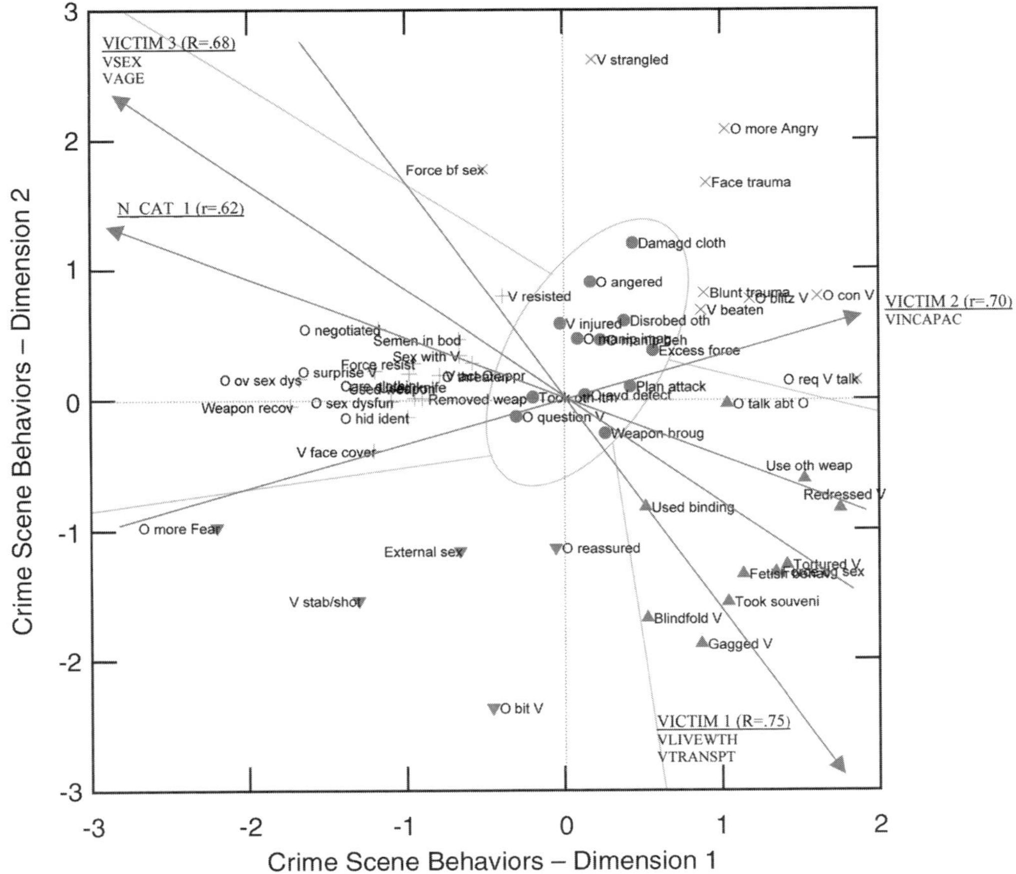

Fig. 7.2. Victim characteristic cluster vectors fitted to the two-dimensional sexual assault crime scene behavior multidimensional scaling coordinates.

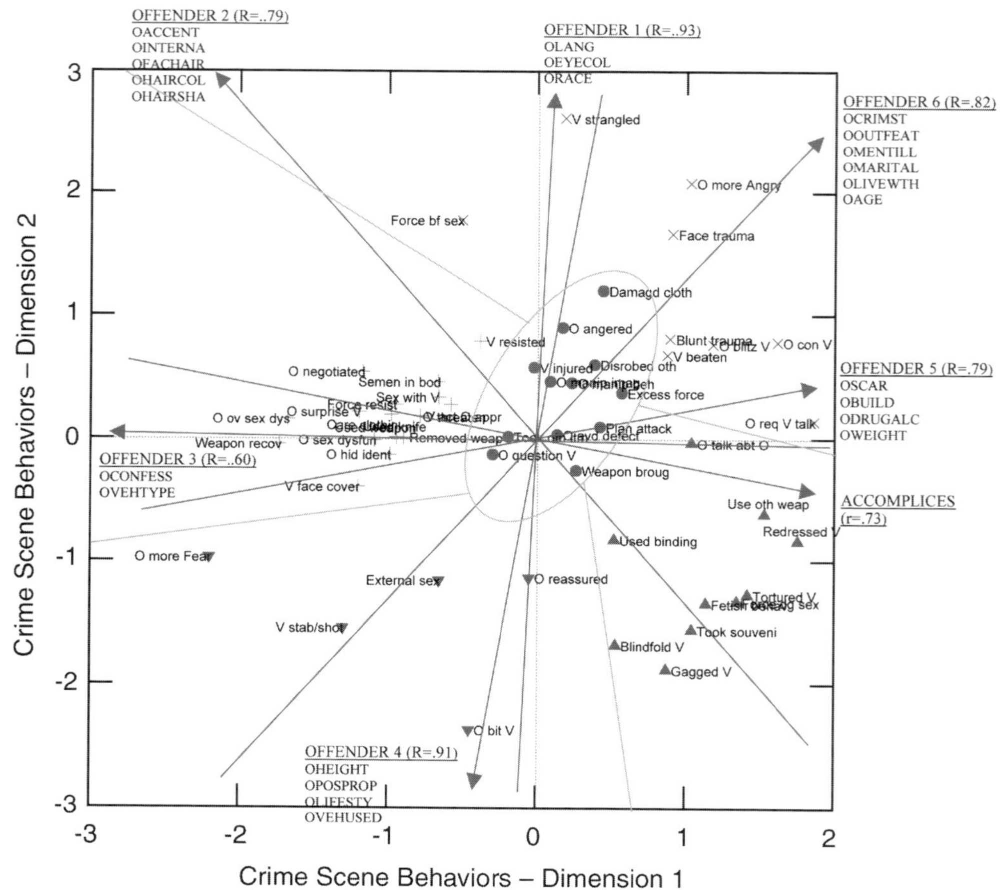

Fig. 7.3. Offender characteristic cluster vectors fitted to the two-dimensional sexual assault crime scene behavior multidimensional scaling coordinates.

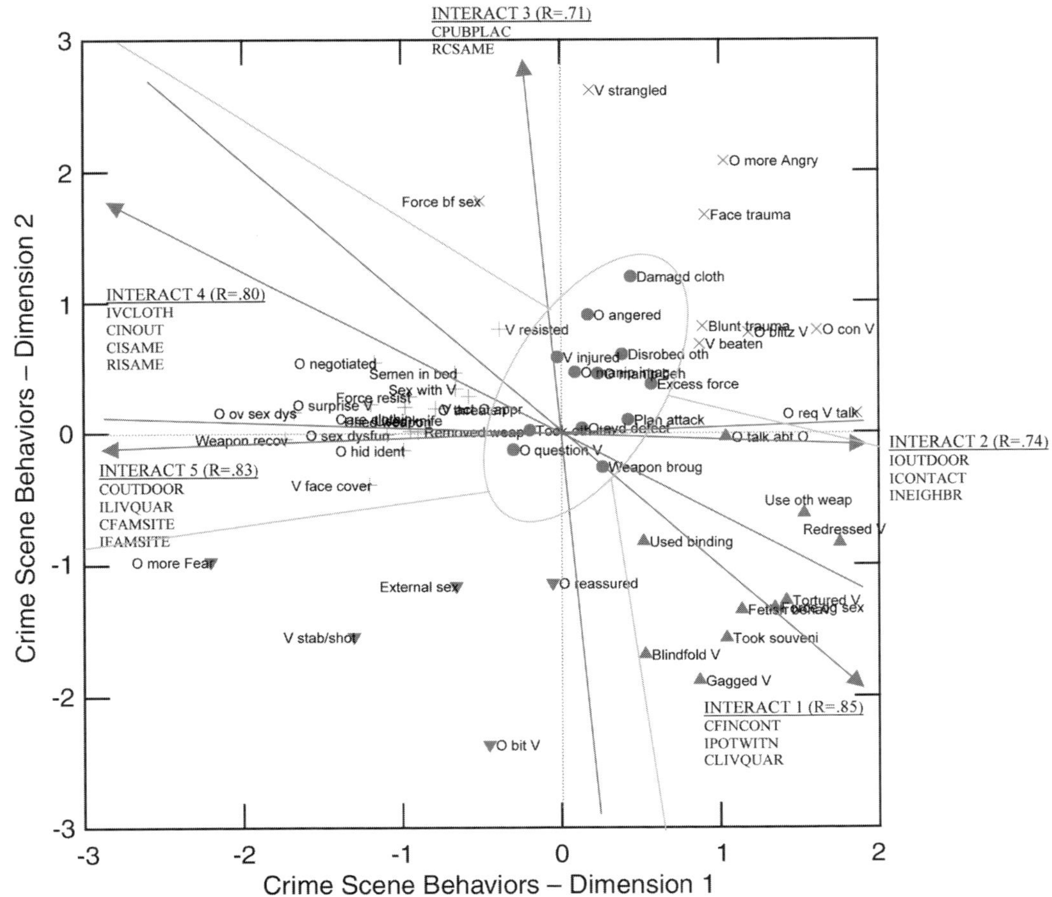

Fig. 7.4. Offender–victim interaction characteristic cluster vectors fitted to the two-dimensional sexual assault crime scene behavior multidimensional scaling coordinates.

offender, and their interaction to facilitate interpretation and understanding of the dimensionality of crime scene behaviors. These analyses explicitly linked crime scene characteristics to conditional probability patterns that would be most useful in profiling offenders and their victims. Previous work by researchers such as Canter and Heritage *(17)*, Knight et al. *(29)*, and Warren et al. *(30)* have provided mostly indirect statistical linkages.

Appendix C contains tables that provide the numerical data (e.g., standardized regression weights and multiple *r* values, averaged dimensional regression weights, and canonical correlations) used to facilitate the property-fitting exercise for the victim, offender, and offender–victim interaction variable sets, respectively. Each table also shows the hierarchical clustering structure associated with each conceptual group of variables and provides the vector cluster labels to be employed in Figs. 7.2–7.4.

Interpretation of Figs. 7.2–7.4 is relatively straightforward, especially when interpreted in conjunction with the regions identified in Fig. 7.1. There is one plot for each of the three conceptual sets of variables. Each fitted vector on a plot summarizes the average relationship that exists between a specific cluster of external characteristics and the two dimensions (i.e., the spatial pattern) of the MDS solution. The strength of the relationship is measured by the canonical correlation between the two dimensional coordinates and the conditional probability scores for the variables in the cluster. The direction of the relationship directly reflects the combination of signs of the averaged standardized regression weights for the two dimensions. Therefore, movement toward the arrowhead for any vector is interpreted as reflecting an increasing tendency (i.e., the conditional probability that the variable takes on a value of 1 when a crime scene characteristic takes on a value of 1); the variables comprising the vector's cluster take on a coded value of 1 when combined with the crime scene characteristics near the arrowhead, and vice-versa when moving toward the tail of the vector.

Victim Characteristics

Figure 7.2 shows the fitted property vectors for the three identified clusters of victim characteristics. The victim 1 vector showed higher conditional probabilities with crime scene characteristics falling into the *ritual* cluster. Thus, there were higher probabilities of victims at crime scenes in which the ritual variables took on a coded value of 1, living with other people and relying on others for their transport. The victim 2 vector suggested a higher probability of victims at crime scenes in which the *brutality* variables took on a coded value of 1, being incapacitated at the time of initial contact. The victim 3 vector revealed higher probabilities of victims at crime scenes in which the *intercourse* variables took on a coded value of 1, being female and 21 years old or older. One additional vector is shown as reflecting a statistically significant fit in Fig. 7.2, namely the vector for one of the two statistical control variables, N_CAT_1. This variable measured the number of instances in the sample of crimes in which each crime scene behavior took on a value of 1 (as defined in Appendix B). The vector clearly shows that the more frequently occurring category 1 crime scene behaviors were found in the *intercourse* cluster, whereas less frequently occurring category 1 crime scene behaviors were found in the *ritual* cluster.

Offender Characteristics

Figure 7.3 shows the fitted property vectors for the six identified clusters of offender characteristics. Also fitted was an offender-related single variable vector, gleaned from the cases addressing whether or not accomplices were involved. The offender 1 vector suggested higher probabilities of offenders at crime scenes in which the *brutality* variables took on a coded value of 1, being bilingual, having darker eye color, and being non-white in racial background. The offender 2 vector revealed higher probabilities of offenders at crime scenes in which the intercourse (spatially, this vector also bordered on the *brutality* region) variables took on a coded value of 1, having an accent, traveled internationally within the last 10 years, facial hair, and darker hair color and shade. The offender 3 vector showed higher probabilities of offenders at crime scenes in which the *intercourse* variables took on a coded value of 1, confessing to other similar crimes of violence and driving an SUV, van, or truck. The offender 4 vector suggested higher probabilities of offenders at crime scenes in which the *chaotic* (spatially, this vector also bordered on the predator region) variables took on a coded value of 1, being taller, in possession of some property from other people, having a criminal lifestyle, and using a vehicle in the crime. The offender 5 vector suggested higher probabilities of offenders at crime scenes in which the *brutality* (spatially, this vector also bordered on the *ritual* region) variables took on a coded value of 1, having a scar, being larger in build, showing evidence of drug or alcohol use, and being heavier in weight. Similarly to the offender 5 vector but more clearly aligned with the *brutality* cluster, the offender 6 vector revealed higher probabilities of offenders at crime scenes in which the *brutality* variables took on a coded value of 1, being on statutory release, having some type of outstanding physical feature, showing evidence of mental illness, living with other people, and being older. The accomplices vector showed an increasing likelihood for accomplices to be involved in crimes in which the *ritual* (spatially, this vector also bordered on the *brutality* region) variables took on coded values of 1. Similarly, the multiple offenders vector showed an increasing likelihood for offenders with a longer series of offenses to be involved in crimes in which the *ritual* variables took on coded values of 1.

Offender–Victim Interactions

Figure 7.4 shows the fitted property vectors for the five identified clusters of offender–victim interaction characteristics. The interact 1 vector suggested higher probabilities of offender–victim interactions at crime scenes in which the *ritual* variables took on a coded value of 1, the contact between the offender and victim was interrupted or the victim escaped, there were potential witnesses in the initial contact area, and the crime scene was in the victim's living quarters. The interact 2 vector revealed higher probabilities of offender–victim interactions at crime scenes in which the *ritual* (spatially, this vector also bordered on the *brutality* region) variables took on a coded value of 1 and the initial contact scene was outdoors and non-residential. The interact 3 vector showed higher probabilities of offender–victim interactions at crime scenes in which the *brutality* variables took on a coded value of 1, the crime scene was in a public place, and the recovery site and crime scene were the same. The interact 4 vector revealed higher probabilities of offender–victim interactions at crime scenes in which the *intercourse* variables took on a coded value of 1, something was done to the victim's clothing at the initial contact site, the crime scene was outdoors, and the initial contact and crime scenes were the same. The interact 5 vector revealed higher probabilities of offender–victim interactions at crime scenes in which the *intercourse* (spatially, this vector also bordered on the *chaotic* region) variables took on a coded value of 1, the crime scene was outdoors, the initial contact site was in the victim's living quarters, and the offender was familiar with both the crime scene and the initial contact site.

Discussion

The data depicted in Fig. 7.1 has yielded an empirically robust model of serial rape behaviors. The central cluster encompassed by the ellipse contains behaviors that are common to all offenses of serial rape. Surrounding this central cluster are four discernible, empirically distinct clusters (or patterns), each of which correlate with distinct offender characteristics (Figs. 7.2–7.4). This analysis therefore yields a model of serial rape behaviors that will allow for the interpretation of serial rape behavior patterns and the prediction of associated offender characteristics—the objective of profiling.

The most central behaviors in serial rape crimes are not those indicative of sexual intercourse, but rather, those associated with the offender's planning and precautions taken to avoid apprehension. This finding questions the coherency of the FBI's organized–disorganized typology being applied consistently to rape *(15)*. The presence of preparatory and precautionary behaviors in the central cluster serves to support the expansion of the organized–disorganized behavior maxim beyond a simple dichotomy and into a more sophisticated continuum. The basic tenet of the dichotomy is the categorical distinction of crime behavior patterns by their level of sophistication. The key measure for this level of sophistication being indications of planning on the part of the offender by, for example, observing precautions to elude apprehension. The presence of precautionary behaviors as a central, commonly occurring theme weakens the categorical distinction of the organized–disorganized dichotomy and suggests that all rape patterns commonly share some level of sophistication and then diverge toward the poles of a conceptual continuum. Thus, patterns to the right in Fig. 7.1 contain behaviors indicative of a higher level of planning and sophistication, whereas those to the left are more indicative of a lower level of premeditation.

Additionally, the observation of precautionary behaviors as a central feature of rape behavior is not fully consistent with the findings of the FBI research on serial rapists *(16)*. Although it supports the conclusion of Hazelwood and Burgess *(16)* that serial rapists predominantly plan their offenses, it appears to conflict with the observation that rapists seldom employ tactics for avoiding apprehension. The position of the behavioral icon "*offender avoid detection*" being located in the central cluster is indicative of this point. Indeed, the proposition that the vast majority of serial rapes are premeditated and yet involve offenders who do not take precautions to avoid apprehension is inconsistent with the fundamental premise of organized behavior. This inconsistency is highlighted by the results in Fig. 7.1.

Also confirming premeditation by way of cluster centrality is the presence of behaviors indicative of robbery, appearing next to the focal aspect of serial rape. Specifically, the offender brings a weapon to the offense, communicates with the victim, and takes items of property (theft). However, it must be noted that although theft occurs as a common behavior among rapists, it may not, as a motivating factor, be the same for each of the outlying behavior clusters. For example, one cluster of rapists may thieve because of anger, another because it represents a further expression of control, another because it is an opportunistic act irrelevant to the reason for the rape.

The final group of behaviors in the central cluster conveys a theme of violence, as seen by the offender's anger, the victim's injury, and the damage caused to the victim's clothing. However, this aspect of violence is, perhaps not surprisingly, a central element to any analysis involving sexual assault. The central themes of rape in the present model therefore are premeditation, robbery, and the expression of violence. This finding raises a number of conceptual questions when considering previous research. In Canter and Heritage's *(17)* model, the central theme of rape was concluded to be the treatment of the victim as a sexual object. However, the present model suggests that planning and perpetration of the offense on the part of the offender with an associated expression of sexual violence forms the basis of most serial rapes. Consequently, the present model seems to suggest elements of both impersonal criminality and the expression of violence. This aspect of violence is in accordance with the propositions of Groth et al. *(14)*. The element of impersonal criminality exemplified by the theme of robbery and premeditation seems more akin to the theory of rape proposed by Rada *(31)* or Scully and Marolla *(20)*. That is, many rapes are simply perpetrated by individuals who carry out numerous criminal acts and for whom rape is one such mode of expressing criminal activity.

Although robbery, violence, and premeditation appear as common behavioral patterns, it seems unlikely that rape is an incidental aspect of these crimes. It would seem a more reasonable conclusion that planning and robberies are a common, integral aspect of rape, with an underlying theme of violence. In this regard, varying degrees of violent behavior can be observed in the outlying patterns.

From an investigative perspective, the base behaviors in the central cluster can be used in the development of criminal profiles via a reductive method. In line with previous literature *(15)*, behaviors located in the central pattern were interpreted as indicative of certain offender characteristics. With the current Fig. 7.1 model, it can be seen that the identification of offender characteristics cannot heavily rely on the presence of these undifferentiated crime behaviors, because these behaviors are common to all patterns of serial rape behavior. Perhaps the only inference that can be drawn from the presence of these undifferentiated behaviors is that the crime can be inferred to be part of a rape series.

Moving to the outlying patterns, cluster 2 or the *brutality* pattern, represents a facet of behaviors demonstrating an explosive release of anger in a sexual assault. Typically in this pattern, the offender uses a confidence trick to lure the victim and then suddenly assaults them in an escalating and excessive fury of blunt force blows and/or strangulation. Violence occurs before any sexual interference and consequently, its evident purpose is not to induce suffering or simple compliance for intercourse, but rather, to achieve degradation and total dominance over the victim. The theme of the behaviors observed in this pattern clearly bear a strong resemblance to the anger pattern described by Groth et al. *(14)*.

Offenders in the *brutality* pattern tend to be relatively older, have scars and a criminal record, and are typically in some form of conjugal relationship. Perhaps this combination of characteristics is not surprising when we consider that an older individual is more likely to accumulate these features through the vicissitudes of life. These offenders tend not to collect souvenirs of their crime and typically do not confess to their activities. This last behavioral feature suggests that these offenses are characterized by a more defiant and resentful mindset.

Cluster 4 continues the theme of violence represented in Fig. 7.1 and is termed the *ritual* pattern. This pattern is indicative of ritualized and paraphilic behavior closely linked with sexual sadism. Indications of planning are clearly visible through behaviors such as binding, gagging, blindfolding, and even torturing the victim. Indeed, in this cluster, the close association of torture, fetishism, and force during sex are noteworthy features. Clearly sexual sadism is an integral aspect of this pattern. Souvenir collection also distinctively occurs and victims tend to be male, and offenses often committed by multiple offenders.

The *ritual* pattern bears a number of interesting similarities to concepts identified by other researchers. Within much of the sexual assault literature, there is a clear association between this behavior pattern and both the sadistic offender pattern proposed by Groth et al. *(14)* and the violence pattern described by Canter and Heritage *(17)*. Additionally, there are clear parallels between the ritual pattern and some typologies found in the literature on sexual/serial murder. Although murder has not occurred, the overall pattern and theme of behaviors in the ritual pattern show a substantial concordance with those of the lust murderer *(23,24,32,33)* or the organized, sadistic offender from the FBI's sexual murder taxonomy *(15,22)*. Namely, offenders are highly rational, well-groomed, and mobile in the commission of their offenses. These strong similarities with the generic lust murderer and the organized offender pattern raise the possibility that this phenomenon represents interrupted sexual murders that for some reason did not result in death. Indeed, the *ritual* pattern may actually represent a phase in the development/evolution of the lust murderer. The *ritual* pattern demonstrates some congruence with behavioral factors found to be indicative of offenders who escalate in violence with subsequent offenses *(34)*. Additionally, inexperienced offenders will be more likely to be interrupted, but eventually may want to indulge in more aberrant violent acts during their offenses, or indeed eliminate the principal witness and thus graduate to murder. This area of speculation draws some support from the current model, where offenses in the *ritual* pattern have a tendency of being interrupted and result in the victim's release or escape.

In contrast to the violence exemplified by the *brutality* and *ritual* patterns occupying the right half of Fig. 7.1, the *intercourse* pattern (i.e., cluster 3) to the left side of the model is a less aggressive, almost passive, form of assault. In this behavior pattern, the main objective of the assault is to have sexual intercourse with the victim. Violence, be it ritualistic or punitive, is simply not an integral part of the assault. The use of force is barely sufficient to secure compliance from the victim. Thus, Fig. 7.1 shows that the offender converses and threatens the victim to achieve control and then proceeds to intercourse.

An interesting factor to emerge from the *intercourse* pattern is that although intercourse seems to be the focal objective of this offender's actions, offenders tend to experience sexual dysfunction. The presence of these two factors seems to be more than mere coincidence. Indeed, the offender characteristics describe almost diminutive, meek individuals, which suggest that these behaviors may represent an attempt by offenders to assert themselves through sexual prowess to compensate for sexual inadequacies experienced in other normal circumstances.

The scenario typified by these offenses seems to involve an invasion of the victim's abode by the offender. Once inside these premises, the offender typically either carries out the entire offense within the home, or moves the victim to another location. In this pattern, offenders generally take precautions to conceal their identity by, for example, wearing a mask or covering the victim's face. Although covering the victim's face in sexual murder has been described as an act of depersonalization in this type of murder *(15)*, in the present model (*see* Fig. 7.1), the close proximity of the offender hiding his or her identity by covering the victim's face seems to suggest that concealment of the offender's identity or a sense of shame over sexual inadequacy may be more likely the motive.

This pattern has a number of conceptual similarities with the findings of previous research. Rather than featuring any overt themes of anger or domination such as those predicted by Groth et al. *(14)*, the *intercourse* pattern demonstrates a style of offense in which intercourse is the focal behavior. This pattern nevertheless mirrors the sexuality facet of rape behaviors observed by Canter and Heritage *(17)* and also concurs with Marshall's *(21)* notion that rape may represent a desire for social contact or intimacy. It is, however, important to note that although the intercourse pattern shares a common theme with Canter and Heritage's *(17)* sexuality pattern, the intercourse exhibited in the current model does not share any other common variables.

The fourth pattern identified in the model is the *chaotic* pattern (i.e., cluster 5). This evidently is marked by an impulsive and violent offense style. In this pattern, the offender performs violent behaviors that are potentially lethal and cruel, and yet these actions in their totality do not convey any sense of coordinated purpose, such as a systematic and sadistic inducement of suffering or an excessively explosive release of violence. Here, the extent of sexual interference/intercourse with the victim is superficial in nature and primarily involves external manipulation such as fondling or digital penetration. Again, it seems that sexual interaction with the victim is more of an opportunistic act, than one involving a premeditated purpose.

Offenders are typically young and consequently are unlikely to have any identifiable features or social patterns that come with age (e.g., scars, tattoos, a partner). However, a distinct feature to note in this pattern is that offenders are highly prone to steal property from the victim. From the combination of crime behaviors and offender characteristics, a tentative scenario begins to emerge that explains this pattern. The *chaotic* pattern seems to represent the actions of a young opportunistic offender who haphazardly embarks on some form of larceny and sexual assault. The offender's age and possible inexperience may explain the violence and general disorder evident in the commission of their crime(s).

The *chaotic* pattern also poses an interesting contradiction when compared with past research. The spontaneous nature of the rape and the level of violence in chaotic interactions are similar to some of the actions of the anger rapist *(14)*, but the underlying theme of such an assault does not seem to reflect any hatred or desire on the part of the offender to dominate the victim. The element of theft in this pattern seems to correspond with the underlying theme of criminal enterprise common to all patterns in this model. Specifically, this pattern also bears some relation to the criminality category of rape identified by Canter and Heritage *(17)*. Thus, the *chaotic* pattern, to some degree, embodies the concept of impersonal criminal actions that are primarily unrelated to rape.

However, a more compelling, conceptual similarity with the *chaotic* pattern can be found in the literature relating to sexual murder. Here, the disorganized offender is characterized by a spontaneous and violent crime style akin to the *chaotic* pattern *(15)*. Thus, the *chaotic* pattern is congruent with the disorganized offender in many respects, with the exception of the offender suffering from a mental disorder. Consequently, the disorganized offense style may be an indication of a sane, youthful, but inexperienced offender, or it may represent the actions of an individual suffering from a mental disorder.

The general themes of the present model appear quite similar to those observed in the sexual murder model discussed in Chapter 8 *(35)*. Patterns observed to the right-hand side of the present model are those associated with a more extreme expression of violence. Thus, the *ritual* pattern resembles the behaviors in the *predator* pattern and *brutality* corresponds with the *fury* pattern of the sexual murder model. Similarly, the *intercourse* pattern concords well with the sexual murder rape pattern, and the *chaotic* pattern matches with the *perversion* pattern. The fact that the general configuration of this model is similar to that observed in sexual murder is an indication of the similarity between behaviors involved in sexually violent crimes.

One explanation for these similarities may lie in the development of offenders from rapists to murderers. That is, offenders may escalate in their level of violence from serial rape to sexual murder. This conceptual pathway has been observed in the previous convictions of sexual killers *(36,37)*. Thus, the results of the present study suggest that offenders can potentially carry their style of offense on to sexual killings and may fulfill a motive or need that is distinct to their specific cluster in this way.

This idea of serial rapists possibly graduating to sexual murder is a concept that warrants greater empirical scrutiny in the future. In the interim, however, the model presented in this chapter, it is hoped, will assist in advancing the quest for further empirically grounded knowledge in the area of criminal profiling for the purpose of better understanding the phenomena of serial rape.

Acknowledgment

This chapter has been amended from material previously published by: Kocsis, R.N., Irwin, H.J., Cooksey, R.W. (2002). Psychological profiling of offender characteristics from crime behaviors in serial rapists. International Journal of Offender Therapy and Comparative Criminology, 46(2), 144–169.

References

1. Oleson, J.C. (1996). Psychological profiling: Does it actually work? Forensic Update, 46, 11–14.
2. Ault, R.L. and Reese, J.T. (1980). A psychological assessment of crime profiling. FBI Law Enforcement Bulletin, 49 (3), 22–25.
3. Berkerian, D.A. and Jackson, J.L. (1997). Critical issues in offender profiling. In: Jackson, J.L. and Berkerian, D.A., eds. Offender profiling: Theory, research and practice. Chichester, UK: Wiley, pp. 209–220.
4. Copson, G., Babcock, R., Boon, J., Britton, P. (1997). Articulating a systematic approach to clinical crime profiling. Criminal Behavior and Mental Health, 7, 13–17.
5. Copson, G. and N. Marshall. (1999). Mind over matter. Police Review, 11 (6), 16–17.
6. Gudjonsson, G., and Copson, G. (1997). The role of the expert in criminal investigations. In: Jackson, J.L. and Berkerian, D.A., eds. Offender profiling: Theory, research and practice. Chichester, UK: Wiley, pp. 61–76.

7. Hormant, R. J. and Kennedy, D. B. (1998). Psychological aspects of crime scene profiling: Validity research. Criminal Justice and Behavior, 25(3), 319–343.
8. Jackson, J.L. and Berkerian, D.A. (1997). Does offender profiling have a role to play? In: Jackson, J.L. and Berkerian, D.A., eds. Offender profiling: Theory, research and practice. Chichester, UK: Wiley, pp. 1–9.
9. Keppel, R.D. and Walter, R. (1999). Profiling killers: A revised classification model for understanding sexual murder. International Journal of Offender Therapy and Comparative Criminology, 43(4), 417–437.
10. Nowikowski, F. (1995). Psychological offender profiling: An overview. The Criminologist, 19(4), 255–273.
11. Oldfield, D. (1997). What help do police need in their inquiries? In: Jackson, J.L. and Berkerian, D.A., eds. Offender profiling: Theory, research and practice. Chichester, UK: Wiley, pp. 93–107.
12. Stevens, J.A. (1997). Standard investigatory tools and offender profiling. In: Jackson, J.L. and Berkerian, D.A., eds. Offender profiling: Theory, research and practice. Chichester, UK: Wiley, pp. 77–93.
13. Wilson, P. and Soothill, K. (1996). Psychological profiling: Red, green or amber? The Police Journal, 119(1), 12–20.
14. Groth, N.A., Burgess, A.W., Holmstrom, L.L. (1977). Rape: Power, anger and sexuality. American Journal of Psychiatry, 134(11), 1239–1243.
15. Ressler, R.K., Burgess, A., Douglas, J.E. (1988). Sexual homicide: Patterns and motives. New York: Lexington Books.
16. Hazelwood, R.R. and Burgess, A.W. (1995). Practical rape investigation: A multidisciplinary approach, 2nd ed. Boca Raton, FL: CRC Press.
17. Canter, D.V. and Heritage, R. (1989). A multivariate model of sexual offence behavior: Developments in offender profiling. I. Journal of Forensic Psychiatry, 1(2), 185–212.
18. Prentky, R.A., Cohen, M., Seghorn, T.K. (1985). Development of a national taxonomy for the classification of rapists: The Massachusetts Treatment Center System. Journal of the American Academy of Psychiatry Law, 13, 39–70.
19. Kocsis, R.N., Irwin, H.J., Hayes, A.F. (1998). Organised and disorganised behaviour syndromes in arsonists: A validation study of a psychological profiling concept. Psychiatry, Psychology and Law, 5(1), 117–130.
20. Scully, D. and Marolla, J. (1983). Incarcerated rapists: Exploring a sociological model. Final report for the Department of Health and Human Services. Tockville, MD: National Institute of Mental Health.
21. Marshall, W.L. (1989). Intimacy, loneliness and sexual offenders. Behavior Research in Therapy, 27, 491–503.
22. Douglas, J.E., Burgess, A.W., Ressler, R.K. (1992). Crime classification manual. New York: Simon and Schuster.
23. Hickey, E.W. (1997). Serial murderers and their victims, 2nd ed. CA: Wadsworth.
24. Holmes, R.M. and Holmes, S.T. (1998). Serial murder, 2nd ed. Beverly Hills, CA: Sage.
25. Hair, J.F. Jr., Anderson, R.E., Tatham, R.L., Black, W. G. (1998). Multivariate data analysis, 5th ed. Upper Saddle River, NJ: Prentice Hall.
26. Kruskal, J.B. and Wish, M. (1978). Multidimensional scaling. Beverly Hills, CA: Sage.

27. Coxon, A.P.M. (1982). The user's guide to multidimensional scaling. London: Heinemann Educational Books.
28. Cohen, J. and Cohen, P. (1983). Applied multiple regression/correlation analysis for the behavioral sciences, 2nd ed. Hillsdale, NJ: Erlbaum.
29. Knight, R.A., Warren, J.I., Reboussin, R., Soley, B.J. (1998). Predicting rapist type from crime-scene variables. Criminal Justice and Behavior, 25(1), 46–80.
30. Warren, J., Reboussin, R., Hazelwood, R.R., Gibbs, N.A., Trumbetta, S.L., Cummings, A. (1999). Crime scene analysis and the escalation of violence in serial rape. Forensic Science International, 100, 37–56.
31. Rada, R.T. (1978). Psychological factors in rapist behaviour. In: Rada, R.T., ed. Clinical aspects of the rapist. NY: Grune and Stratton, pp. 21–58.
32. Brown, J.S. (1991). The psychopathology of serial sexual homicide: A review of the possibilities. American Journal of Forensic Psychiatry, 12(1), 13–21.
33. Revitch, E. and Schlesinger, L. B. (1989). Sex murder and sex aggression: Phenomenology, psychopathology, psychodynamics and prognosis. IL: Charles C. Thomas.
34. Warren, J., Reboussin, R., Hazelwood, R., Cummings, A., Gibbs, N., Trumbetta, S. (1998). Crime scene and distance correlates of serial rape. Journal of Quantitative Criminology, 14(1), 35–59.
35. Kocsis, R.N., Cooksey, R.W., Irwin, H. J. (2002). Psychological profiling of sexual murders: An empirical model. International Journal of Offender Therapy and Comparative Criminology, 46(3), 532–553.
36. Ressler, R.K., Burgess, A.W., Douglas, J.E., Hartman, C.R., D'Agostino, R.B. (1986). Sexual killers and their victims: Identifying patterns through crime scene analysis. Journal of Interpersonal Violence, 1(3), 288–308.
37. Ressler, R.K., Burgess, A.W., Hartman, C.R., Douglas, J.E., McCormack, A. (1986). Murderers who rape and mutilate. Journal of Interpersonal Violence, 1(3), 273–287.

Chapter 8

Criminal Profiling of Sexual Murder Offenses

Summary

This chapter reports on the study of sexual murder offenses for the purpose of profiling similar crimes in the future. The study involved the analysis of 85 cases of sexual murder using multidimensional scaling. The analysis of these cases produced a five-cluster model of sexual murder behavior. First, a central cluster of behaviors was identified that represent behaviors common to all patterns of sexual murder. Next, four distinct outlying patterns, entitled predator, fury, perversion, and rape, were identified each demonstrating distinct offense styles. Further analysis of these patterns also identified distinct offender characteristics.

Key Words: Sexual/serial murder; criminal profiling.

INTRODUCTION

Analogous to the previous chapter concerning the profiling of serial rape offenses and despite the evident popularity of criminal profiling in general, surprisingly few original, quantitative, academically reviewed studies have been published that examine crimes of sexual murder for the specific purpose of criminal profiling. Possibly the most cited original study in the area of sexual murder profiling or profiling in general for that matter, was by the FBI's Behavioral Science Unit *(1)*. This study reported on the analysis of 36 incarcerated sexual murderers within North America. This research resulted in the organized–disorganized behavior dichotomy. The underlying premise of this dichotomy is the interpretation of crimes by their level of behavioral sophistication and corresponding offender characteristics. Thus, the organized category represents a methodical, premeditated crime with corresponding offender

From: *Criminal Profiling: Principles and Practice*
By: R. N. Kocsis © Humana Press Inc., Totowa, NJ

characteristics such as maturity, resourcefulness, and typically sexual perversion. Inversely, the disorganized category represents a haphazard, almost random crime with the corresponding inverse offender characteristics of immaturity, opportunism, and the likelihood of some mental disorder *(1)*.

Although this study has attracted considerable citation and discourse, empirical replications of this research have been lacking. One of the few empirical replications of this dichotomy was by Kocsis et al. *(2)*. The findings of this research revealed that the concept of interpreting crimes by their level of behavioral sophistication holds some merit. However, a more realistic interpretation of crime behaviors requires development beyond a simple dichotomous categorization. Future research should aim to construct a model that will allow for the scientific and objective interpretation of crime behaviors and associated offender characteristics.

Aside from these few empirical studies, the literature on sexual murder profiling is dominated by various proposed offender taxonomies. The foremost of these being the FBI's *Crime Classification Manual (3)*, which uses the organized–disorganized dichotomy as a basis for classifying sexual murder. The limitations of this dichotomy, however, are in some way acknowledged by the development of a further intermediary category known as the mixed offender. Additionally, the proposal of another new category, called the sadistic offender, seems to be already encapsulated within the parameters of the organized offender.

In the sexual murder typologies proposed by Holmes and Holmes *(4)* and Hickey *(5)*, common characteristics are identifiable among the offender categories identified by the work of the FBI. The Holmes' categories rely primarily on the inference of offender motivations and associated psychogenic factors. Similarly, the Hickey categories are based on a combination of inferred motivations with demographic features, such as the offender's gender, sexual orientation, and the use of accomplices.

The typologies of both Holmes and Holmes *(4)* and Hickey *(5)* commonly identify an offender category delineated by a pattern of selection of unknown victims with physical and sexual assault being perpetrated on such victims for psychological gain. Holmes describes this gain as similar to sexual sadism (*4*, p. 62), whereas Hickey favors goals of power and control with sexual sadism as a subsidiary drive (*5*, p. 154). This common offender category identified by Holmes and Holmes *(4)* is encapsulated under the broad title of hedonism with its subcategories of lust and thrill killers. Similarly, Hickey *(5)* refers to this pattern as men who kill women (based on the predominant gender pattern of these offenses). Hickey, however, also assigns the lust killer label to this category. Thus, common themes of anger, intercourse, and sadism seem to be discernible from the various sexual murder typologies.

Both Holmes and Holmes *(4)* and Hickey *(5)* also elaborate on various other sexual murderer categories that are distinguished primarily by the murder of multiple victims. Here, a number of highly diverse categories are propounded. The motivations for these categories include such factors as political beliefs, histrionic attention, or monetary gain. Such a vast diversity of categories poses problems for the conceptualization and coherent understanding of sexual murder as Chapter 5 has already discussed. That chapter proposed a more focused definition of sexual murder in which offenders can be identified by an underlying composite of psychological components as opposed to an overinclusive definition of serial crime.

In addition to the literature on sexual murder profiling, the material on sexual assault profiling is also relevant to the further development of a scientific, objective model of sexual murder profiling. The first body of relevant work is by Groth et al. *(6)*. The central thesis of this study is that rape represents the sexually violent expression of power and domination rather than an act of sexual desire. Two broad categories of rapist motivation are offered: power rape, in which the offender's primary motivation is power and control over the victim, and anger rape, in which the offender's primary motivation is an expression of hatred and contempt for the victim.

Work has also been undertaken by the FBI's Behavioral Science Unit into rape profiling *(7)*. The starting point of this unit's work was the adoption of the offender categories proposed by Groth *(8)*. However, for the purpose of developing information that would be directly relevant to the needs of law enforcement, a study of incarcerated North American serial rapists was also undertaken. This study resulted in the compilation of an extensive list of serial rape demographic information.

Finally, Canter and Heritage *(9)* offer five categories of sexual assault behavior: intimacy (in which intimacy is attempted with the victim), sexuality (in which intercourse is the crucial element in the assault), violence (in which the attack is characterized by violent action), impersonal (in which the victim is treated as an object), and finally criminality (in which the assault is not overtly sexual in nature). As outlined in Chapter 7, the research of Canter and Heritage *(9)* is different from previous literature on sexual assault in that their categories are based exclusively on the empirical analysis of offender actions. The basic hypothesis of profiling is that offenders differ in their actions and that these differences in behavior relate to the offender's characteristics. Consequently, the interpretation of crime actions requires the classification of offense behaviors as distinct from any inferred motivation. On this score it is argued by Canter and Heritage *(9)* that previous studies on profiling, such as those undertaken by Groth et al. *(6)*, which combine inferred motivations with actions, are empirically flawed. A further methodological aspect arising from the research of Canter and Heritage *(9)* concerns the distinct empirical discrimination between varying crime behaviors. One criticism of previous studies is that some have made no allowances for the possibility of commonalties in behavior among the various offender typologies, whether in the crime of sexual assault or murder.

The objective of the study in this chapter was to undertake an empirical analysis of crime actions, distinct from inferred motivations, in a sample of sexual murder crimes. Additionally, the selection of cases for this study employed the criteria for sexual murder discussed in Chapter 5 and thus avoided any potentially confounding surplus of cases. It was envisaged that the analysis would result in the development of an empirical model of sexual murder behavior comprising distinct behavior clusters. Furthermore, these empirically distinct behavior clusters could be analyzed to identify associated offender characteristics. The direct statistical matching of behaviors to offender characteristics using this form of analysis had, until this point, never been undertaken. The literature had instead been characterized by qualitative associations between offender behaviors and offender characteristics. Additionally, the present study aimed to identify potential behaviors that are nondiscriminatory, and thus commonly observable in all behavior patterns of sexual murder.

METHOD

Data Pool and Data Screening Process

The study consisted of 85 murder cases from 1960 to 1998 whose characteristics fitted the general pattern of sexual murder discussed in Chapter 5. All offenders in the sample had been convicted of at least one sexual murder and the case history for each was held by various police jurisdictions. Many cases had missing details on numerous variables. Frequency distributions were computed for all variables in the data pool. The goal was to achieve a stable and internally consistent data pool comprising variables of sufficient non-missing entries as well as sufficient variability across the categories within each variable. Variables presenting largely constant data values were removed before analysis, as were variables that were missing across a large portion (i.e., more than 50%) of the data pool.

Variable Condensation

To facilitate data analysis and interpretation, conceptually similar categories for each variable were collapsed to produce dichotomous (0, 1) measures having a reasonable number of category 1 responses. Most variables were recoded on a presence–absence basis, whereas others were recoded into less–more-type categories. Some variables having multiple categories were dummy coded into several dichotomous variables (e.g., the variables for initial contact location, crime scene location, recovery site location, type of weapon used, etc.). Variables with very few or no category 1 responses were deleted with the exception of the burning [*V burned*] variable (n = 2 category 1 responses).

As a result of this data screening and variable condensation process, some 260 variables were reduced to the final set of 137 variables employed in the study. Variables were broadly grouped into conceptual sets for subsequent analyses: victim characteristics (14 variables), offender characteristics (36 variables), offender–victim interaction characteristics (22 variables), and crime scene characteristics (65 variables). All variable labels and extended names used for the multidimensional scaling (MDS) diagrams are shown in Appendix D.

Analysis Process

The analysis consisted of several steps. The first step involved a nonmetric MDS analysis of the 65 dichotomous crime scene characteristics to identify the appropriate number of dimensions, ranging from two- to five-dimensional solutions, to interpret *(10)*. This analysis was accomplished with the MDS program in SYSTAT 7.0 using the Guttman coefficient of alienation minimization criterion and the Jaccard measure of binary similarity.

The second step involved a cluster analysis of the resulting MDS coordinates to facilitate a regional interpretation of the dimensional solution *(11)*. Ward's minimum variance method of clustering was employed for this step using the squared Euclidean distance measure of dissimilarity. The dimensional coordinates of the MDS solution were standardized (converted to z-scores), then plotted on a scatterplot using cluster identifiers to differentiate the plotting symbols.

The third step in the analysis involved fitting the external property vectors, using variables from the victim, offender, and offender–victim interaction variable sets, to the MDS coordinates for each of the 65 crime scenes. For this step, a new data pool was created containing the standardized dimensional coordinates from the MDS analysis and conditional probabilities for each characteristic variable not used in the MDS analysis. Each conditional probability was found as the mean of the external variable of interest within the category coded 1 for a specific crime scene characteristic. This mean was, in effect, the conditional probability that the variable (e.g., victim's sex [VSEX]) equaled 1 (female) when a specific crime scene characteristic (e.g., unpatterned wounds [UNPATTER]) also equaled 1 (unpatterned wounds were present). These conditional probabilities became the external characteristic property vector variables that were to be fitted to the MDS coordinates to aid in its interpretation. For statistical control purposes, two additional new variables were created that indicated the number of non-missing cases (out of 85 cases) for each crime scene variable and the number of observations comprising the category coded as 1 for each crime scene variable.

Property fitting was accomplished using an extension of the multiple regression procedure for fitting direction cosines described by Kruskal and Wish (*11*, pp. 87–88). Each of the conditional probability variables within a specific conceptual set (e.g., victim characteristic set, offender characteristic set, and offender–victim interaction characteristic set) were predicted from the standardized MDS coordinates using the set correlation analysis procedure in SYSTAT 7.0 (*see* ref. *12*, for a discussion of set correlation as a multivariate relational technique). Both the predictor set (MDS coordinates) and criterion set (conditional probability variables) were partialled for the influence of the number of non-missing observations and for the number of observations comprising the category coded as 1 to control for the possible influences of missing data and small category 1 membership. The appropriate multivariate canonical correlation, associated with each variable set comprising the cluster for each vector, was recorded and tested for overall significance.

Working from the univariate level, each significant external characteristic variable with a set was identified (based on the omnibus F-test for the regression analysis of that variable). Then, the standardized regression coefficients for each of the MDS dimensions for each significant variable within the set of interest were cluster-analyzed using Ward's method with the Euclidean distance measure and the most appropriate number of clusters of characteristics then identified. For each such identified cluster, the standardized regression weights for each dimension were averaged across the variables comprising the cluster.* On separate MDS dimensional plots (one for each conceptual set of variables analyzed), the external characteristic property vectors for each

*To illustrate the first few steps of the property-fitting process, consider the steps taken to analyze the variables in the victim characteristics set. The 14 variables comprising this set were individually regressed onto the two standardized MDS

cluster of variables were fitted using the averaged regression β weights, which were transformed to yield a specific vector angle that was then drawn onto the graph with an arrowhead. The angle computed ranged between 0 and 360° and thus directly indicated the direction in which the association arrowhead should point.†

RESULTS

Multidimensional Scaling

After closely examining each of the two- through five-dimensional solutions, the two-dimensional solution was identified as most appropriate for interpretation (coefficient of alienation = 0.264; $R^2 = 0.758$). The higher order dimensional solutions, although producing marginally better data fit, were conceptually difficult to clearly interpret. Interpretability was the ultimate criterion to be met by the solution adopted. Figure 8.1 shows the plot of the standardized coordinates for the two-dimensional MDS solution for the 65 crime scene characteristics.

---

* (*continued from opposite page*) dimension coordinates and the resulting standardized (β) weights for the two dimensions were recorded (thus 14 distinct regression were run for this set—although the set correlation method in SYSTAT ran them all simultaneously). Out of the 14 original variables in the set, only the victim's marital status (VMARITAL) was not significantly predicted by the MDS coordinates and was therefore dropped from further consideration. The remaining set of weights (13 variables by two weights) was cluster-analyzed and three distinct clusters of variables were identified. One such cluster comprised the VRACE, VLIVEWTH, and VINCAPAC variables and the standardized weights for each dimension were averaged across the three, giving average β weights for dimensions 1 and 2. These two averaged weights then formed the basis for fitting the property vector to the two-dimensional MDS solution plot.

† The specific formulas used for this transformation were as follows where *a* and *b* reflect the two dimensions that anchor the graph in question:

$$if(\beta_a > 0 \text{ and } \beta_b > 0)\ \text{angle} = \deg\left[(\cos^{-1}\beta_a / \sqrt{\beta_a^2 + \beta_b^2})\right]$$

$$if(\beta_a > 0 \text{ and } \beta_b < 0)\ \text{angle} = 360 - \deg\left[(\cos^{-1}\beta_a / \sqrt{\beta_a^2 + \beta_b^2})\right]$$

$$if(\beta_a < 0 \text{ and } \beta_b > 0)\ \text{angle} = 180 - \deg\left[(\cos^{-1}|\beta_a| / \sqrt{\beta_a^2 + \beta_b^2})\right]$$

$$if(\beta_a < 0 \text{ and } \beta_b < 0)\ \text{angle} = 180 + \deg\left[(\cos^{-1}|\beta_a| / \sqrt{\beta_a^2 + \beta_b^2})\right]$$

The two-dimensional MDS coordinates were hierarchically clustered and five clusters of crime scene characteristics were identified. These five clusters divided the two-dimensional space of crime scene characteristics into five non-overlapping regions. The five clusters of coordinates are marked by distinct plotting symbols in Fig. 8.1 (the cluster regions have also been drawn in). Figure 8.1 could be interpreted several ways, but a regional interpretation is one of the clearest. Crime scene characteristics appearing in the same region of the plot were inspected for common themes to arrive at an interpretation of what each region might be indicating.

The central cluster 1 (surrounded by the ellipse) represented crime scene characteristics that were not clearly discriminated by the two-dimensional MDS structure—they were associated by virtue of having similar coordinate patterns centered on or near zero for each dimension. Thus, these particular crime scene characteristics were not very useful for distinguishing between different crime scenes in the sense of anything uniquely meaningful about the crime scene. The four regions surrounding the central regions represented distinct clusters of crime scene characteristics that tended to appear together sufficiently often to constitute a distinctive pattern.

Cluster 5, to the right of the central ellipse, seemed to capture a pattern of very violent crime scene characteristics suggesting an element of deliberateness and cruelty in the behaviors. The cluster 5 region suggested a *predator* pattern. Cluster 4, to the left of the central ellipse, seemed to capture crime scene characteristics suggestive of less violent intent in which the offender and victim tended to be acquainted and brutality was not strongly evident—almost as if the death had not been intended. Cluster 4 suggested a *rape* pattern. Cluster 3 suggested a pattern of crime scene behaviors that had a very violent nature but with much less calculation and deliberation being evident, perhaps coupled with a motive of revenge—an anger theme seemed to underscore this region. Thus, cluster 3 seemed to clearly identify a *fury* pattern. Finally, cluster 2 captures crime scene behaviors suggestive of an antisocial perversion theme but without the calculation evident in cluster 5. Cluster 2 therefore suggested a *perversion* pattern.

External Property Vector Fitting

Figures 8.2 to 8.4 summarize the property vector-fitting analyses designed to explicitly relate clusters of the characteristics of the victim, the offender, and their interaction to facilitate interpretation and understanding of the dimensionality of crime scene behaviors. These variables are considered external properties because they were not used to generate the MDS solution. These analyses explicitly link crime scene characteristics to conditional prob-

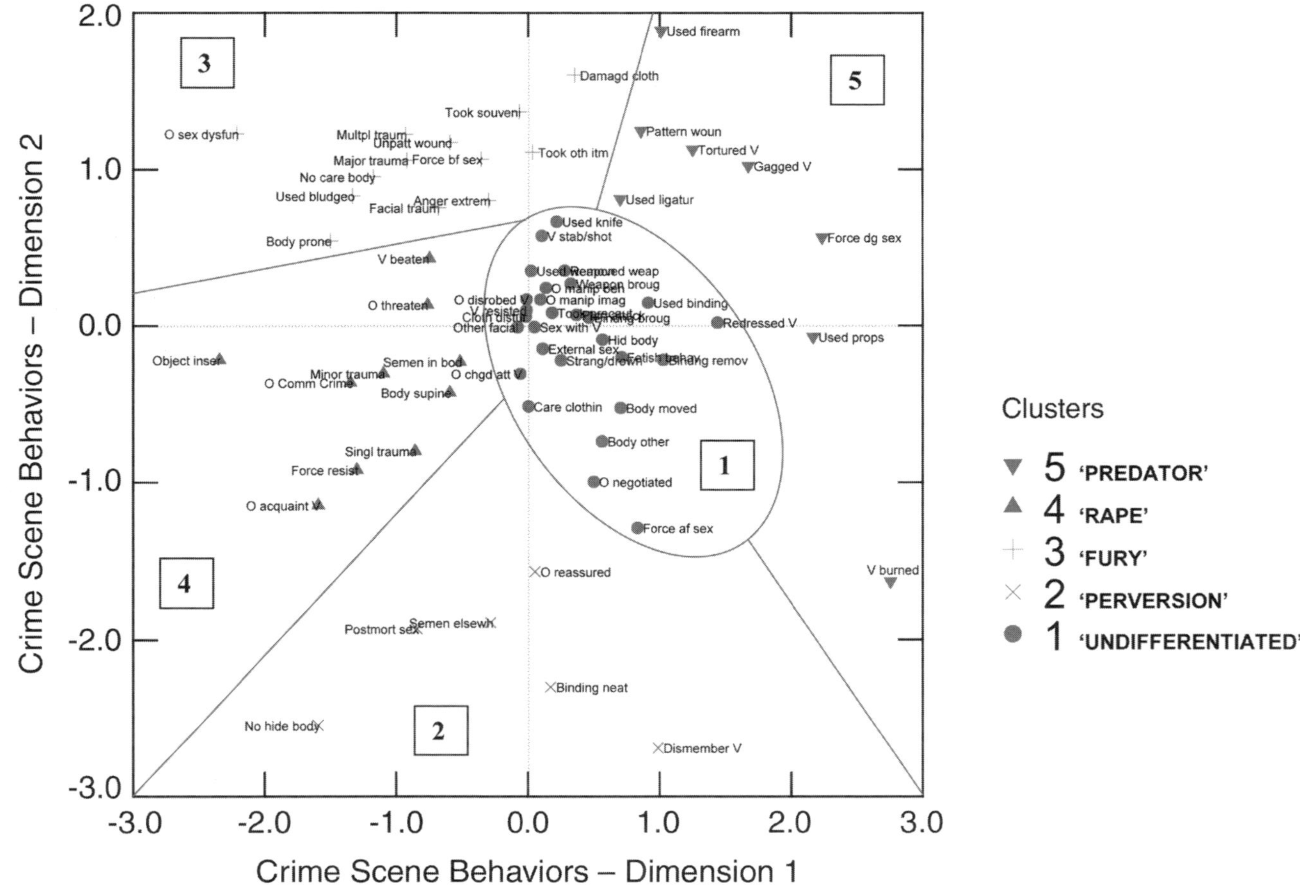

Fig. 8.1. Two-dimensional murder crime scene behavior multidimensional scaling solution with coordinate cluster structure superimposed.

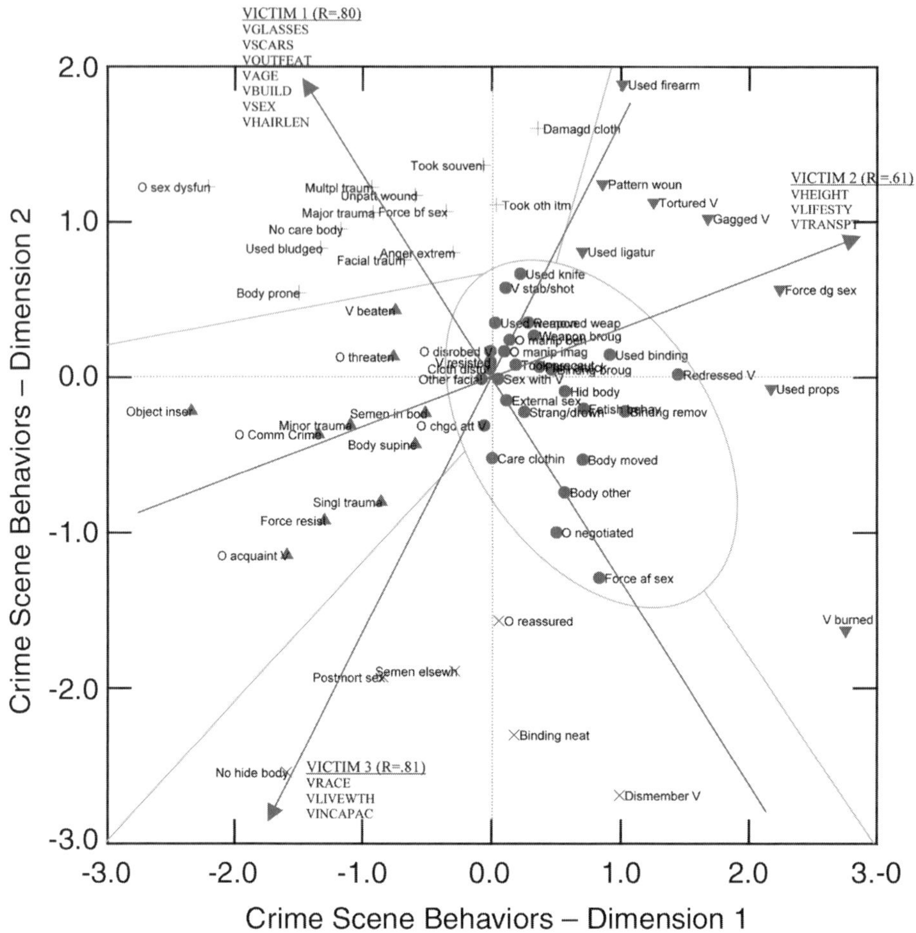

Fig. 8.2. Victim characteristic cluster vectors fitted to the two-dimensional murder crime scene behavior multidimensional scaling coordinates.

ability patterns that are most useful in profiling offenders and their victims. This sort of direct statistical linkage has not, to the author's knowledge, been made concrete within the context of a single database in previous research. The tendency has been to scale both crime scene behaviors and offender and victim characteristics in separate MDS analyses, and then make conceptual and qualitative arguments as to how the various scaling patterns might relate *(9)*. In contrast, Knight et al. *(13)* employed a somewhat different non-pattern-based bootstrapping methodology to predict rapist types from crime scene variables using two unrelated data sets.

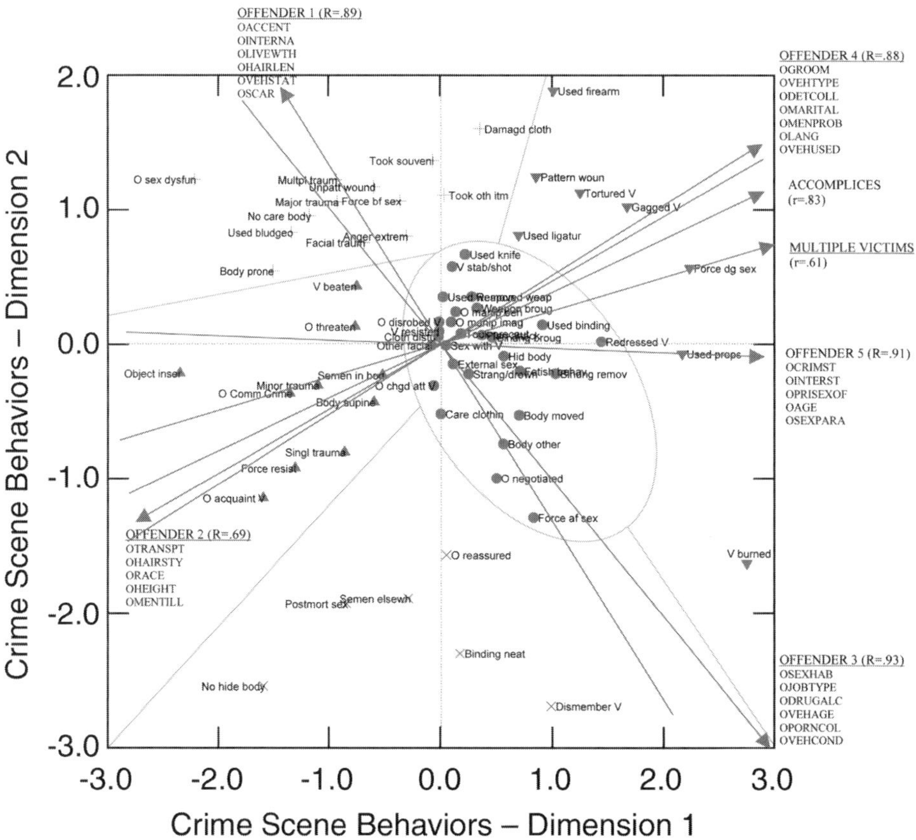

Fig. 8.3. Offender characteristic cluster vectors fitted to the two-dimensional murder crime scene behavior multidimensional scaling coordinates.

Appendix E contains tables that provide the numerical data (e.g., standardized regression weights and multiple *r* values, averaged dimensional regression weights, and canonical correlations) used to facilitate the property-fitting exercise for the victim, offender, and offender–victim interaction variable sets, respectively. Each table also shows the hierarchical clustering structure associated with each conceptual group of variables and provides the vector cluster labels to be employed in Figs. 8.2 to 8.4.

Interpretation of Figs. 8.2 to 8.4 is relatively straightforward, especially when interpreted in conjunction with the regions identified in Fig. 8.1. There is one plot for each of the three conceptual sets of variables. Each fitted vector on a plot summarizes the average relationship that exists between a specific cluster of external characteristics and the two dimensions (i.e., the spatial

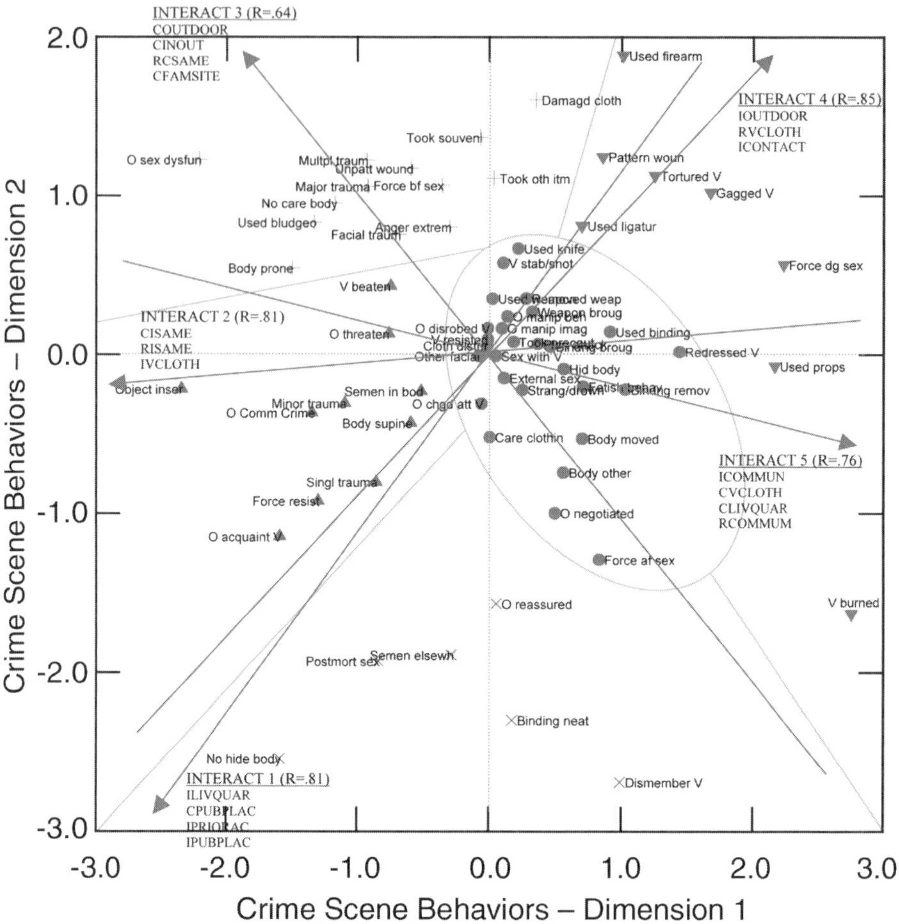

Fig. 8.4. Offender–victim interaction characteristic cluster vectors fitted to the two-dimensional murder crime scene behavior multidimensional scaling coordinates.

pattern) of the MDS solution. The strength of the relationship is measured by the canonical correlation between the conditional probability scores for the variables in the cluster and the two-dimension coordinates. The direction of the relationship directly reflects the combination of signs of the averaged standardized regression weights for the two dimensions. Thus, movement toward the arrowhead for any vector is interpreted as reflecting an increasing tendency (i.e., the conditional probability that the variable takes on a value of 1 when a crime scene characteristic takes on a value of 1) for the variables comprising the vector's cluster to take on a coded value of 1 in conjunction with the crime scene characteristics near the arrowhead, and vice versa when moving toward the tail of the vector.

Victim Characteristics

Figure 8.2 shows the fitted property vectors for the three identified clusters of victim characteristics. The victim 1 vector showed higher conditional probabilities with crime scene characteristics falling into the *fury* cluster. Thus, there were higher probabilities of victims wearing glasses, having scars or other marks or outstanding features, being older and of larger build, being female, and having longer hair length at crime scenes where the *fury* variables took on a coded value of 1. The victim 2 vector suggested higher probabilities of victims being taller, having a more criminal lifestyle, and relying on others for their transportation at crime scenes where the *predator* variables took on a coded value of 1. The victim 3 vector revealed higher probabilities of victims being non-white, living with others, and being incapacitated in some form at the time of initial contact at crime scenes where the *perversion* variables took on a coded value of 1.

Offender Characteristics

Figure 8.3 shows the fitted property vectors for the five identified clusters of offender characteristics. Also fitted were two offender-related single variable vectors, gleaned from the 65 case files, addressing whether or not accomplices were involved along with the offender in the crime and the number of offenses committed by the offender identified for each crime. At crime scenes where the *predator* variables took on a coded value of 1, the offender 1 vector suggested higher probabilities of offenders having an accent, having traveled internationally within the last 10 years, living with others, having longer hair length, not owning their vehicles, and having scars or other identifying marks. At crime scenes where the *rape* variables took on a coded value of 1, the offender 2 vector revealed higher probabilities of offenders relying on others for their transportation, having an unkempt hair style, being non-white, being taller, and showing evidence of mental illness. At crime scenes where the *perversion* variables took on a coded value of 1, the offender 3 vector showed higher probabilities of offenders having homosexual/bisexual tendencies, being employed, showing evidence of drug/alcohol use, driving an older vehicle, having a collection of pornography, and having a vehicle in exceptionally good condition (spatially, this vector bordered on the predator region as well). At crime scenes where the *predator* variables took on a coded value of 1, the offender 4 vector suggested higher probabilities of offenders being well-groomed, driving a van/SUV/truck, owning a collection of detective magazines, being married, having a history of mental problems, being bilingual, and using a vehicle in the crime. Similar to the offender 4 vector, at crime scenes where the *predator* variables took on a coded value of 1, the offender 5 vector revealed higher probabilities of offenders being on statutory release, having traveled interstate within the last 10 years, having a history of prior sex offenses, being older, and having a collection of sexual paraphernalia. The accomplices vector showed an increased likelihood for accomplices to be involved in crimes in which the *predator* variables took on coded values of 1. Similarly, the multiple victims vector showed an increased likelihood for offenders with a longer series of offenses to be involved in crimes in which the *predator* variables took on coded values of 1.

Offender–Victim Interactions

Figure 8.4 shows the fitted property vectors for the five identified clusters of offender–victim interaction characteristics. At crime scenes where the *perversion* variables took on a coded value of 1, the interact 1 vector suggested higher probabilities of offender–victim interactions in which the initial contact was in the victim's living quarters, the crime scene in a public place, a history of prior offender activity in the initial contact area, and initial contact in a public place (spatially, this vector bordered on the rape region as well). At crime scenes where the *rape* variables took on a coded value of 1, the interact 2 vector revealed higher probabilities of offender–victim interactions in which the crime scene and initial contact scene were the same, the recovery site and the initial contact site were the same, and in which something had been done to the victim's clothing at the initial contact site. At crime scenes where the *fury* variables took on a coded value of 1, the interact 3 vector showed higher probabilities of offender–victim interactions in which there was an outdoor crime scene/site, the same crime scene and the recovery site, and in which the offender was unfamiliar with the crime site. At crime scenes where the *predator* variables took on a coded value of 1, the interact 4 vector revealed higher probabilities of offender–victim interactions in which there was an outdoor initial contact site and something was done to the victim's clothing at the recovery site. Similarly, at crime scenes where the *predator* variables took on a coded value of 1, the interact 5 vector revealed higher probabilities of offender–victim interactions in which the initial contact was in a non-city location, something was done to the victim's clothing at the crime scene, the crime scene was in the victim's living quarters, and the recovery site was in a non-city location.

Conclusion

The results depicted in Fig. 8.1 represent an attempt to present empirically a coherent model of sexual murder behaviors. The central cluster (undifferentiated behaviors) indicates behavior common to all offenses of sexual murder. Surrounding this central cluster are four empirically different patterns of behavior, each correlating with distinctive offender characteristics (Figs. 8.2–8.4). Consequently, this model allows for the interpretation of murder behavior patterns and the identification of probable offender characteristics associated with each of the discerned behavior patterns.

Three key themes appear to characterize the behaviors in the central cluster: intercourse with the victim, violence, and premeditation/precaution in the perpetration of the offense. The incidence of sex and violence is perhaps unsurprisingly a central theme of sexual murder and concurs with the commonly cited drives for sexual murder *(4,5)*. Indeed, this combination of sexuality and violence also concurs with the basic premise by Groth et al. *(6)* for sexual assault. However, the exact relationship between these two themes (i.e., whether the primary theme is the expression of violence and control through sexuality or vice versa) is indeterminable. Given that the victim dies during the encounter, it could be inferred that violence and force are indeed primary factors.

The presence of preparatory and precautionary behaviors in the central undifferentiated cluster supports the expansion of the organized–disorganized behavior maxim beyond a simple dichotomy and toward instead a more sophisticated continuum. The basic premise of the dichotomy is the categorical distinction of crime behavior patterns by their level of sophistication. The key measure for this level of sophistication are indications of planning for the offense, such as undertaking precautions to elude apprehension. The presence of preparation/precautions as a central theme weakens this categorical distinction and indicates that all patterns commonly share some level of sophistication and then diverge out toward the poles of a conceptual continuum.

The undifferentiated behaviors also assist in the construction of profiles via a reductionist process. In line with previous literature *(1)*, behaviors located in this central pattern were interpreted as indicative of certain offender characteristics. For example, the use of restraints or the removal of a weapon were identified as being key features of an organized offender and from this conclusion various organized offender characteristics were espoused *(1)*. With the current model, it can be seen that identification of offender characteristics cannot rely on the presence of these undifferentiated crime behaviors because these actions are common to all patterns of sexual murder behavior. Perhaps the only inference that can be made from the presence of these undifferentiated behaviors is that the crime can be inferred to be a sexual murder.

In considering the outlying behavior patterns in Fig. 8.1, there are a number of conceptual similarities with previous research literature on sexual murder. Demonstrating the highest level of behavioral congruence is the *predator* pattern. This pattern shares many similarities with the hedonist killer proposed by Holmes and Holmes *(4)*, the lust killer by Hickey *(5)*, and the archetypal organized or sadistic offender of the FBI *(1,3)*: a sexually sadistic predator who tortures and rapes the victim for pleasure.

The description of a hedonist killer given by Holmes and Holmes *(4)* loosely correlates with the predator pattern. However, the subdivision made by Holmes and Holmes into the thrill and lust categories is based on the presence or absence of postmortem sexual activity. Unfortunately, the current model identifies postmortem sexual activity as part of the *perversion* pattern. Consequently, the current model does not support the subcategorization devised by Holmes and Holmes *(4)* in this regard. Speculation that the *perversion* pattern may represent the lust category would be ill-conceived, because this pattern holds many features that are highly incompatible with the broad conception of hedonistic offenders.

Offender characteristics for the *predator* pattern accord well with the existing literature. Offenders are typically older, mobile, living with a partner, and from a white racial background. They are well-groomed and are typically collectors of crime literature and sexual materials and are highly prone to re-offend. However, offenders in the *predator* pattern exhibit a high tendency to operate with an accomplice. Here a significant quandary arises as to how this result may relate to Hickey's *(5)* distinction between team offenders, who are described as being driven by different psychological imperatives, influences, and considerations, and the subcategory of male solo killers (also known as lust killers). Both categories are equally well-catered for by the *predator* pattern and consequently serve to question this distinction.

In the previously discussed literature, the presence of souvenir or token collection behaviors indicates an offender who exhibits the *predator* pattern *(3–5)*. However, in the current model, souvenir and token collection features are exhibited in the adjacent *fury* pattern. Irrespective of the statistical classification of these behaviors within the *fury* pattern, they appear in a close bordering proximity to the *predator* pattern. This suggests that although these behaviors are statistically distinguished as being within the *fury* pattern, they can nonetheless appear to be associated with the *predator* pattern when adopting a broad directional interpretation of the model in contrast to the present regional clusters.

The *fury* pattern represents an explosive, unfocused obliteration of the victim. A number of similarities exist between the *fury* pattern and existing literature. The excessive uncoordinated violence and overall disorganization characteristic of this pattern demonstrates a similarity to the visionary killer espoused by Holmes and Holmes *(4)* or the archetypal disorganized offender category espoused by the FBI in its organized–disorganized dichotomy. However, there is the implicit assumption in both categories that the actions are the product of an individual operating under some form of psychotic delusion. The present results, however, indicate that there is an equal propensity for offenders to suffer from, or not to suffer from, a mental disorder. Consequently, although a portion of offenders within the *fury* pattern may be identified as violent and mentally ill, an equal portion of offenders are unlikely to suffer from any such disorder. This obviously conflicts with the visionary or disorganized offender hypothesis.

An alternative interpretation of the *fury* pattern can be deduced from the literature on sexual assault and specifically the anger retaliation rapist espoused by Groth et al. *(6)*. The anger retaliation rapist is described as a non-psychotic offender who possesses an irrational, deep hatred that is expressed as a violent sexual assault. If this category were extended into the domain of murder, in which the offender's assault kills the victim, it would plausibly explain the non-psychotic element in the *fury* pattern. Indeed, this rational, but hateful offender hypothesis could explain the retention of souvenirs or trophies in the *fury* pattern. The taking of such items may remind the offender of their retribution or an added act of defilement and hatred.

In contrast to the general theme of violence exhibited in the *predator* and *fury* patterns, the *rape* pattern represents an offender primarily pursuing intercourse with only the use of force necessary to perpetrate the assault. Consequently, the victim is threatened for compliance and force is only applied to achieve control. This application of force is typically minimal with a few wounds inflicted on the victim's body. There is no indication of sexual dysfunction with penetration occurring and semen usually found in the victim. This pattern therefore seems to resemble a sexual assault that has resulted in murder. Indeed, it is open to speculation as to whether murder was the original intention of the offender or an outcome of the offense. For example, in attempting to control the victim, the offender may deliver a blow that kills the victim. The crime scene behaviors and associated offender characteristics may not demonstrate any great degree of perversion or sadism, but rather, a simple brutal pursuit of intercourse.

Indeed, a unique feature of this pattern is that offenders often have some prior acquaintance with the victim. This does not necessarily imply a prior relationship between the victim and offender but rather, that the offender was aware of the victim's existence before the offense. Interaction characteristics of this pattern indicate that these offenses typically occur in a single indoor location. Through the combination of all of these features, a general scenario for this pattern emerges in the form of a single offender pursuing intercourse and invading a victim's home. The offense is not planned, but more characteristic of an impetuous younger individual who discovers a potential victim and perhaps acts on an impulse of lust and/or desire.

The *rape* pattern represents another challenge to *previous* literature because it is difficult to associate this pattern with any of the homicide categories described by Holmes and Holmes *(4)* or Hickey *(5)*. The pattern coincides with the behavioral principles of a disorganized offender, however, the disorganized category does not adequately explain the observable behavior themes. The closest link to the *rape* pattern stems from the literature on sexual assault. In line with the categories of Groth et al *(6)*, the rape pattern exhibits many facets of the power assertive rapist in pursuing sexual gratification for internal reassurance. Concurrently, the primary behavioral theme of pursuing intercourse also bears a similarity to the sexuality category of rapist identified by Canter and Heritage *(9)*.

Finally, a unique combination of factors comprises the *perversion* pattern. Virtually all crime behaviors in this pattern are related to extreme paraphilic/perverse activity. In contradiction to these perversities, however, offenders are noted to engage the victim in conversation by offering reassurance. Various factors operating in combination explain this pattern. Victims in this pattern typically tend to be younger and male, whereas offenders tend to be older with bisexual or homosexual orientations. The combination of these offender and victim characteristics indicates that these offenses typically involve some form of pedophilic assault that results in the murder of the victim. What may be the motive for the final murder of the victim is contentious. Although this behavior pattern demonstrates passivity in comparison to the violence observed in other patterns, the behaviors present in this pattern are planned and consequently indicate that the murder of the victim is an intentional feature of the assault. Given that this pattern is adjacent to the *predator* pattern, it appears ritualism is a component of the offense. Hickey *(5)* describes a specific category of offender who specializes in the murder of children. The characteristics of the *perversion* pattern match the behaviors and offender characteristics of this type of offender in a way that suggests some form of variant lust killer of children.

In conclusion, the results indicate that sexual murder involves a relationship between sexual activity and violence. However, the exact dynamics behind these two themes remain elusive. Whether sexual murder offenses actually represent serious rape offenses that have escalated in violence and result in the victim's demise is debatable. The very occurrence of the rape pattern in the present model is an indication of such an association. However, in sharp contradiction are the behaviors of the *predator* and *fury* patterns in which the victim's death is an integral element of the offense. Developing a better understanding of the relationship between serial rape and sexual murder will involve a closer study of serious rape offenses.

The empirical model for sexual murder discussed in this chapter can be used for profiling offenses of this nature in the future. This model offers a direct empirical link between crime behaviors and offender characteristics, which is another form of analysis that appears lacking in previous research. This model differs from previous attempts to construct offender typologies that lack empirical structure and which therefore limit their suitability for quantitative comparisons. With the present model as the foundation, it is hoped that further research aiding in the development of sexual murder criminal profiling will occur and progress to the point of a systematic and structured science.

ACKNOWLEDGMENT

This chapter is sourced from material previously published by Kocsis, R.N., Cooksey, R.W., Irwin, H.J. (2002). Psychological profiling of sexual murders: An empirical model. Int J Offender Ther Comp Criminol, 46(3), 532–552.

REFERENCES

1. Ressler, R.K., Burgess, A., Douglas, J.E. (1988). Sexual homicide: Patterns and motives. New York: Lexington Books.
2. Kocsis, R. N., Irwin, H. J., Hayes, A. F. (1998). Organised and disorganised behaviour syndromes in arsonists: A validation study of a psychological profiling concept. Psychiatry, Psychology and Law, 5, 117–130.
3. Douglas, J.E., Burgess, A.W., Burgess, A.G., Ressler, R.K. (1992). Crime classification manual. New York: Simon & Schuster.
4. Holmes, R.M. and Holmes, S.T. (1998). Serial murder, 2nd ed. Newbury Park, CA: Sage.
5. Hickey, E.W. (1997). Serial murders and their victims, 2nd ed. Fresno, CA: Wadsworth.
6. Groth, N.A., Burgess, A.W., Holmstrom, L.L. (1977). Rape: Power, anger and sexuality. American Journal of Psychiatry 134(11), 1239–1243.
7. Hazelwood, R.R. and Burgess, A.W. (1987). An introduction to the serial rapist research by the FBI. FBI Law Enforcement Journal, 56(9), 16–24.

8. Hazelwood, R.R. and Burgess, A.W. (1995). Practical rape investigation: A multidisciplinary approach, 2nd ed. Boca Raton, FL: CRC Press.
9. Canter, D.V. and Heritage, R. (1989). A multivariate model of sexual offence behaviour: Developments in "offender profiling." International Journal of Forensic Psychiatry, 1(2), 185–212.
10. Hair, J.F. Jr., Anderson, R.E., Tatham, R.L., Black, W.G. (1998). Multivariate data analysis, 5th ed. Upper Saddle River, NJ: Prentice Hall.
11. Kruskal, J.B. and Wish, M. (1978). Multidimensional scaling. Beverly Hills, CA: Sage.
12. Cohen, J. and Cohen, P. (1983). Applied multiple regression correlation analysis for the behavioral sciences (2nd ed.). Hillsdale, NJ: Erlbaum.
13. Knight, R.A., Warren, J.I., Reboussin, R., Soley, B.J. (1998). Predicting rapist type from crime-scene variables. Criminal Justice and Behavior, *25*(1), 46–80.

Chapter 9

Criminal Profiling of Serial Arson Offenses

Summary

The practice of criminal profiling is frequently seen as being applicable to crimes of serial arson, although there appears to be little empirical research that examines serial arson offense behaviors in the specific context of criminal profiling. The present study seeks to develop an empirical model of serial arsonist behaviors that can be systematically linked with probable offender characteristics. Analysis has produced a model of offense behaviors that identify four discrete behavior patterns, all of which share a constellation of common nondiscriminatory behaviors. The inherent behavioral themes of each of these patterns are explored in this chapter with discussion of their broader implications for our understanding of serial arson.

Key Words: Serial arson; criminal profiling.

INTRODUCTION

The practice of and research into criminal profiling has predominantly been focused on crimes of sexual violence, such as murder and rape. Although comparatively little research has actually been developed, profiling is nonetheless frequently cited as being also applicable to the investigation of arson crimes *(1–3)*. The objective of the study canvassed in this chapter was to develop an empirical model for the criminal profiling of serial arson offenses.

The majority of current social science research on arson is dominated by psychiatric/psychological studies, which examine issues of mental status and/or offender etiology *(4–8)*, or criminological studies, which either propose varying motive-based classification taxonomies *(9,10)* or anecdotal case studies

(11–13). Despite this body of literature on the broad topic of arson, little empirical material exists on the criminal profiling of arson crimes for criminal investigations, and there is even less on the specific topic of profiling serial arsonists.

Possibly the first and largest body of research to examine arson for the specific purpose of criminal profiling was undertaken by the FBI's Behavioral Science Unit *(14–16)*. The central theme of this research was the development of various motive categories that were correlated with crime behaviors and typical offender characteristics. These studies culminated in the proposal of six broad motive categories for arson *(17)*.

The first category identified, *vandalism*, is described as being motivated by wanton destruction. Offenders are typically juveniles and their crimes demonstrate little sophistication. The second category, *excitement*, deals with motives of psychological stimulation and includes crimes committed for histrionic/heroic desires, to satisfy sexual fetishes, or as a result of psychotic delusion. Offenders in this category tend to be older and such crimes are typically characterized by perpetrators remaining at the crime scene, engaging in masturbation, and the ignition of low-risk targets such as dumpsters and vegetation. The third category, *profit*, deals with arsons motivated by some material gain and frequently involves fraudulent insurance claims by the offender–victim. As the title implies, the fourth category, *revenge*, is committed "in retaliation for some injustice, real or imagined, perceived by the offender" (*17*, p. 173). A prior relationship between the victim and the offender typically characterizes these offenses and there is often evidence of premeditation and planning combined with the use of accelerants. Offenders are typically adult males in blue-collar jobs. The fifth category, *crime concealment*, identifies arson as a means of concealing the evidence of another crime. The sixth and final category, *extremist*, refers to fires that are set to further some social, political, or religious objective.

Perhaps the first study to advance any theory-driven development of profiling techniques for arson was undertaken by Kocsis et al. *(18)*. This study examined the organized–disorganized behavior dichotomy developed by the FBI's Behavioral Science Unit for sexual murderers within the context of arsonists. As indicated in the previous two chapters, the underlying premise of the organized–disorganized dichotomy is the interpretation of sexual murder crime scenes by their level of behavioral sophistication and matching offender characteristics *(19)*.

Although the organized–disorganized typology was developed from a study of sexual murderers, its generalization to arson profiling is evident in the exposition offered by Douglas et al. (*17*, p. 166). The absence of any empirically derived data to support this generalization prompted the study by

Kocsis et al. *(18)*. Within the confined parameters of two forms of arson offenses, this study was able to replicate the dichotomous distinction of the organized–disorganized typology. The results of this study suggested that such a simple dichotomy could not validly be supported when applied to the full gamut of possible behaviors and motivations involved in arson offenses.

A key factor of previous profiling studies, such as Douglas et al. *(17)*, has been the combination of inferred motivations with identifiable behaviors for the construction of the proposed typologies. However, as Canter and Heritage *(20)* indicate, the basic tenet of profiling is that offenders differ in their actions and these differences in behavior relate to the offender's characteristics. Thus, the interpretation of crime actions requires the classification of offense behaviors as distinct from any inferred motivations. Consequently, the majority of studies used for profiling that combine the inference of motivations with observable behaviors are arguably empirically limited.

One previous study that addressed this methodological issue within the context of arson profiling was that of Canter and Fritzon *(21)*. This study identified four basic patterns to arsonist crime scene behavior. The first pattern, labeled *instrumental person*, is described as being the result of some form of dispute between the offender and victim and is reminiscent of a revenge motivation scenario. Characteristics of this pattern include a pattern of threats and arguments between the offender and victim, premeditation in the commission of the offense, and a specific target selected for attack. The second pattern, labeled *instrumental object,* is an opportunistic style of offense with no coherent purpose for the commission of the crime. Behaviors characterizing this pattern include theft of property and fire occurring in an external, visible location typically on a weekday. This pattern was found to be strongly associated with multiple juvenile offenders.

The third pattern entitled *expressive person* is characterized by some form of histrionic goal of the offender with fires being set to "alleviate distress by seeking attention" (*21*, p. 82). Characteristic behaviors in this pattern include the presence of suicide notes with the offender frequently presenting as a victim. The final pattern, labeled *expressive object*, is distinguished by multiple offenses believed to be committed to achieve some form of emotional relief. Behaviors inherent to this pattern include multiple offenses being perpetrated on hospitals, businesses, or public buildings with offenders being triggered into offending by a nonspecific event and remaining at the crime scene to observe the fire.

Although Canter and Fritzon *(21)* make an interesting contribution to the development of arson profiling in general, a number of issues require further investigation to fully inform our understanding of arson, and serial arson profiling in particular. The specific topic of serial arson profiling has been the focus of little empirical research despite the difficulties such offenses present to investigators. Indeed, the technique of profiling has often been found to be of far more utility in the investigation of recidivistic offenses because non-recidivistic crimes can typically be solved by regular investigative procedures *(22)*. This issue in particular serves as an especial impetus for more detailed scrutiny of serial arson crimes.

Irrespective of the crime modality, the majority of profiling studies fail to recognize and account for possible commonalties in criminal behavior. That is, previous studies typically employ categorical typologies that do not allow for the discrimination of a specific pattern of offense from behaviors that may simply be typical of the crime. Additionally, these categorical constructs typically do not provide any impression of the overall relationship between varying categories or any possible co-morbidity of motives between patterns. These are important issues because the actual practice of profiling for criminal investigation purposes does not adopt such static approaches. The published literature on which the practice is supposedly based does not concord with these rigid constructs *(23–25)*.

The present study therefore sought to develop an empirical model for the criminal profiling of serial arson crimes by independently analyzing offense behaviors, thus avoiding the methodological pitfalls of previous studies. Additionally, this analysis set out to distinguish the existence of any common behaviors from those indicative of a specific pattern of behavior. The model developed from the study was expected to provide some understanding of the potential relationships between patterns. Finally, the sample for this study specifically focused on serial arsonists.

METHOD

Data Pool and Data Screening Process

The data pool used in this study consisted of 148 cases of arson from the years 1980 to 1998. All cases satisfied the criteria for serial violent crime as described in Chapter 5. All offenders in the sample had been convicted and incarcerated for their offenses. The variables for this study were extracted from those originally developed by Kocsis et al. *(18)*. These variables were screened and marked for retention in subsequent analysis if they demonstrated sufficient non-missing entries and variability across categories within each variable. Frequency distributions were computed for all variables in the data pool. Extremely small variances (indicating a near constant) were deleted before analysis, as were variables having missing values in more than 50% of data pool cases.

Condensation of the Variables

To facilitate analysis and interpretation, conceptually similar categories for each variable were collapsed to produce dichotomous (0, 1) measures having a reasonable number of category 1 responses. Most variables were recoded on a presence–absence basis, whereas others were recoded into less–more-type categories. Some variables having multiple categories were dummy coded into several dichotomous variables (e.g., variables for arson target, distance offender traveled to target, point(s) of origin for the fire, etc.). Variables with very few or no category 1 responses remaining after this coding process were deleted from the data pool. Several variables were nearly perfectly correlated with other related variables in the data pool and to avoid problems with extreme multi-collinearity, these redundant variables were also deleted from the analysis.

The data screening and variable condensation process yielded a final set of 71 variables. For the major analyses, variables were broadly grouped into conceptual sets: offender personal characteristics (personal set, containing 12 variables), general offender behavior characteristics (general set, containing 14 variables), arson event-specific offender behavior and choice characteristics (event-specific set, containing 16 variables, including 7 variables coding the time and season chosen for the arson event), and crime scene characteristics (crime scene set, containing 29 variables, including variables coding the target of the arson event). A list of these variables is provided in Appendix F.

Analytical Process

The analysis proceeded in several discrete stages commencing with a non-metric multidimensional scaling (MDS) analysis of the 29 dichotomous variables in the crime scene set. This analysis was accomplished using the MDS program in SYSTAT 9.0. Guttman's coefficient of alienation minimization criterion was employed to control the scaling process and Jaccard's measure of binary similarity was employed as the similarity measure. The two-dimensional MDS solution that emerged from this stage was retained for further analysis and interpretation. However, for the purposes of MDS, 29 objects would be considered a sufficient sample for scaling *(26)*.

The second stage of analysis subjected the resulting MDS dimensional coordinates to cluster analysis to facilitate a regional interpretation of the dimensional solution *(27)*. Dissimilarity was measured using the squared Euclidean distance and the clustering algorithm employed was Ward's minimum variance hierarchical method. The standardized dimensional coordinates of the MDS solution were then plotted on a scatterplot using different symbols to distinguish cluster groupings and facilitate identification of crime scene attribute regions. The number of entities clustered in this analysis could be considered as a sufficient sample of serial arsonists for the purposes of cluster analysis *(26)*.

The third stage of analysis focused on fitting external property vectors, using variables from the personal, general, and event-specific variable sets, to the MDS coordinates for each of the 29 variables in the crime scene set. This was accomplished by building up a new data pool containing the standardized coordinates for the two MDS dimensions and conditional probabilities for each dichotomous external property variable not contained in the crime scene set (i.e., those variables contained in the personal, general, and event-specific sets). For a combination of a specific external property variable and crime scene characteristic, the mean for that external property variable within the category coded 1 for that specific crime scene characteristic was computed. This mean directly represented the conditional probability that the external property variable of interest (e.g., OLANG [offender language]) equaled 1 when a specific crime scene characteristic (e.g., TOCCUPY [target was occupied with people at the time of the arson]) also equaled 1. These conditional probabilities defined the external property vector variables statistically fitted to the MDS coordinates.

Property fitting was accomplished using an extension of the multiple regression procedure for fitting direction cosines described by Kruskal and Wish (*28*, pp. 87–88) and implemented in the SYSTAT 9.0 using the Vector method in the perceptual mapping procedure. (Essentially, the procedure was that each external property vector served as a dependent variable in a regression analysis in which the two MDS coordinates served as predictors.) Screening for external property variables that were significantly predicted by the two-dimensional MDS configuration of crime scene characteristics occurred on a variable-by-variable basis. The significance decision was based on the omnibus F-test for the regression analysis of that variable; only those external property vectors that were predictable based on a criterion of $p < 0.05$ were retained for display and interpretation. The final significant external property vectors were displayed in sets by superimposing the fitted vectors (of standardized unit length) in a series of two-dimensional MDS scatterplots. The direction of each vector is defined by the direction and magnitude of the standardized regression coefficient for each of the two MDS dimensions. The fitted vector thus indicates where the relevant external attributes will tend to reflect a code of 1 when the crime scene variables in that region of the MDS space also tend to reflect a code of 1 (i.e., the vector points to where the conditional probabilities are highest).

RESULTS

Multidimensional Scaling

Each of the two- through five-dimensional MDS solutions were examined and the two-dimensional solution was chosen as most interpretable (coefficient of alienation = 0.230; $R^2 = 0.816$). Higher dimensional solutions produced a marginally better fit to the data but at the cost of much greater interpretive complexity and increased noncomparability to previous research findings, such as those in the previous two chapters. Figure 9.1 shows the plot of the standardized coordinates for the two-dimensional MDS solution for the 29 variables in the crime scene set.

The two-dimensional MDS coordinates were hierarchically clustered and five clusters (two of which had meaningful embedded subclusters) of crime scene variables were identified. These clusters divided the two-dimensional space of crime scene variables into five nonoverlapping regions and two subregions. The five clusters of coordinates are marked by distinct plotting symbols in Fig. 9.1 (the cluster regions have also been sketched in); a dotted ellipse and region boundary denotes the meaningful subregion structure. Figure 9.1 could be interpreted in several ways, but a regional interpretation is one of the clearest ways. Crime scene variables appearing in the same region of the plot were inspected for common themes to achieve an interpretation of what each region might be indicating.

The central cluster 1 (surrounded by the solid-boundary ellipse) represented crime scene variables that were not clearly differentiated by the two-dimensional MDS structure—they were associated by virtue of having similar coordinate patterns centered on or near zero for each dimension. Consequently, this cluster was labeled as the common behavior pattern. However, it is clear that within this central region a substructure was identified by the cluster analysis, differentiated somewhat along MDS dimension 1. The small, dotted ellipse surrounds those crime scene variables, separating them from the remaining central variables. The pattern suggests a planned arson event (PLANNED) in which the target was related to the offender (TRELATIO) and physical evidence was left by the offender at the scene (EVIDENCE). This leads to a suggestion that dimension 1 may be connotating some element of closeness or meaningfulness to the offender as well as an element of premeditation, an interpretation that is supported by patterns in other regions more removed from the center.

Premeditation especially seems defensibly suggested by the patterns of variables moving from right to left along dimension 1. Crime scene variables

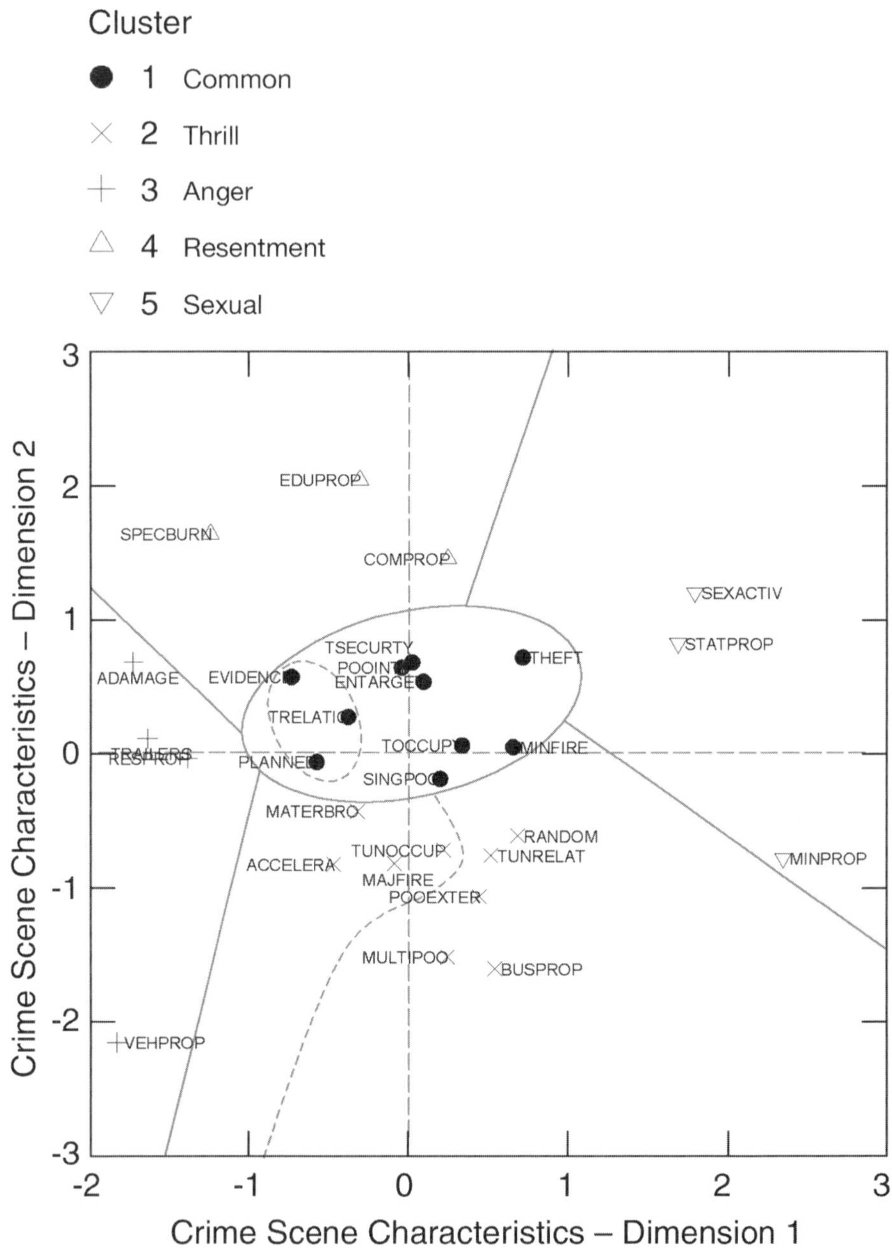

Fig. 9.1. Multidimensional scaling of the crime scene variables in two dimensions with regional hierarchical clustering of scaling coordinates superimposed.

toward the extreme left reflect many aspects associated with a deliberate and planned arson event, bringing materials (MATERBRO), using accelerants (ACCELER) and trailers (TRAILERS), burning specific items (SPECBURN), and deliberate damage to other target items (ADAMAGE). Variables captured in the region of cluster 3 seem to especially reflect a deliberate and directed rage, perhaps of a more personal nature because residential properties and vehicles are the targets included in this cluster. Variables toward the right end of dimension 1 suggest a more random and anonymous arson crime pattern, with a suggestion of disturbance or perverseness (THEFT and SEXACTIV).

The central region is marked by complete omission of presence of any targeted property variables. Inspection of Fig. 9.1 seems to indicate that a major thrust of dimension 2 is to differentiate target properties that were large and public institutions (EDUPROP, STATPROP, COMPROP toward the top of the figure—positive coordinates) from those that were small and noninstitutional (VEHPROP, MINPROP, BUSPROP toward the bottom of the figure—negative coordinates). (RESPROP is at the zero point along dimension 2). The variables captured in the region of cluster 4 seem to be especially related to specific targeted destruction of educational and commercial properties in which specific items are used to start the fires. The suggestion here might relate to a pattern of a strong grudge and directed anger against large public institutions. The region defined by cluster 2 has a defined substructure, differentiated along dimension 1 where the four variables (MATERBRO, ACCELER, TUNOCCUP, and MAJFIRE) to the left of the dotted line are more closely aligned with deliberate planned arson that results in large fires but in unoccupied, smaller-scale properties. Those variables to the right of the dotted line in cluster 2 are more suggestive of unplanned random arson events having multiple and exterior points of origin (MULTIPOO and POEXTER). Targets here tend to be outdoors (BUSPROP and MINPROP) and unrelated to the offender (TUNRELAT). In general, cluster 2 is differentiated from clusters 1, 4, and 5 (toward the opposing end of dimension 2) on the basis of size and institutional nature of the property target, involving a physical man-made structure to destroy (toward the positive pole of the dimension), as well as by the unprotected general nature of the targets in which access is relatively easy (toward the negative pole of the dimension). Note, for example, that the crime variables linked to having to enter the target (ENTARGET), where a security system is present (TSECURTY), single point of entry (SINGPOO), as well as property types being educational, commercial, or state-owned, all suggest protected man-made targets that one has to

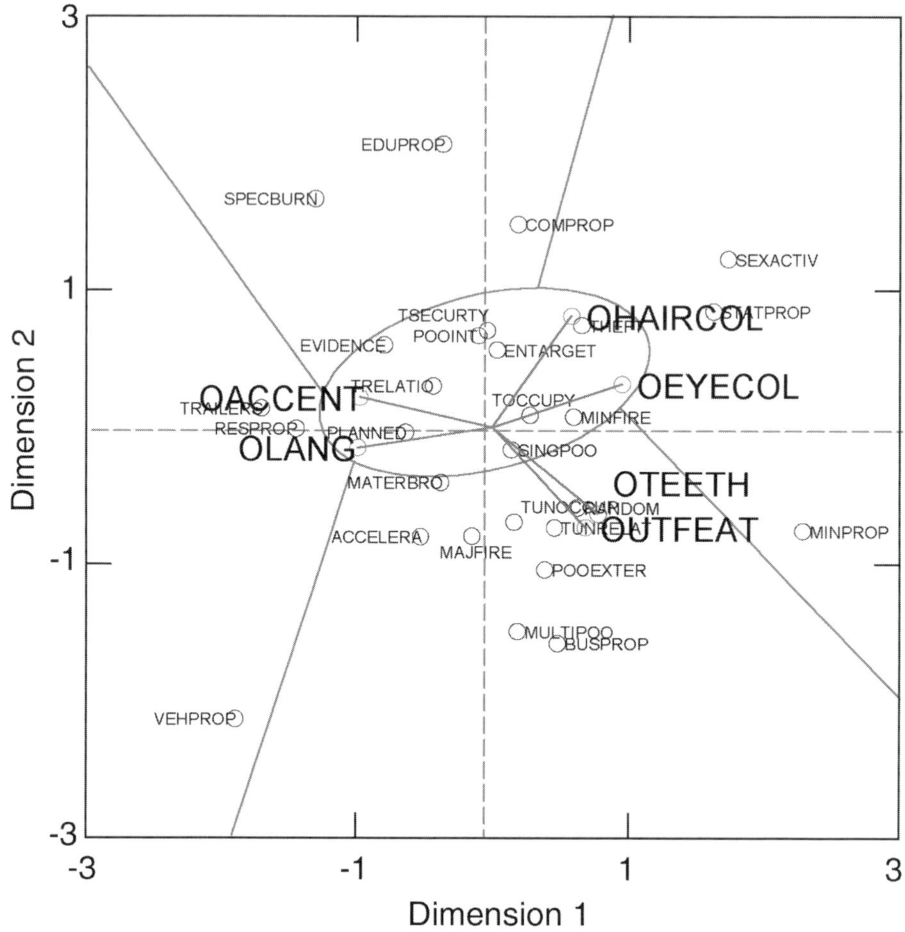

Fig. 9.2. Fitted (significant) personal offender characteristic pattern vectors.

gain access to in order to start a fire—features not captured in the cluster 2 region.

External Property Vector Fitting

Figures 9.2 through 9.4 summarize the property vector-fitting analyses designed to explicitly employ specific characteristics in the personal, general and event-specific variable sets to facilitate interpretation and understanding of the dimensionality of crime scene characteristics. These analyses explicitly link crime scene characteristics to conditional probability patterns that would

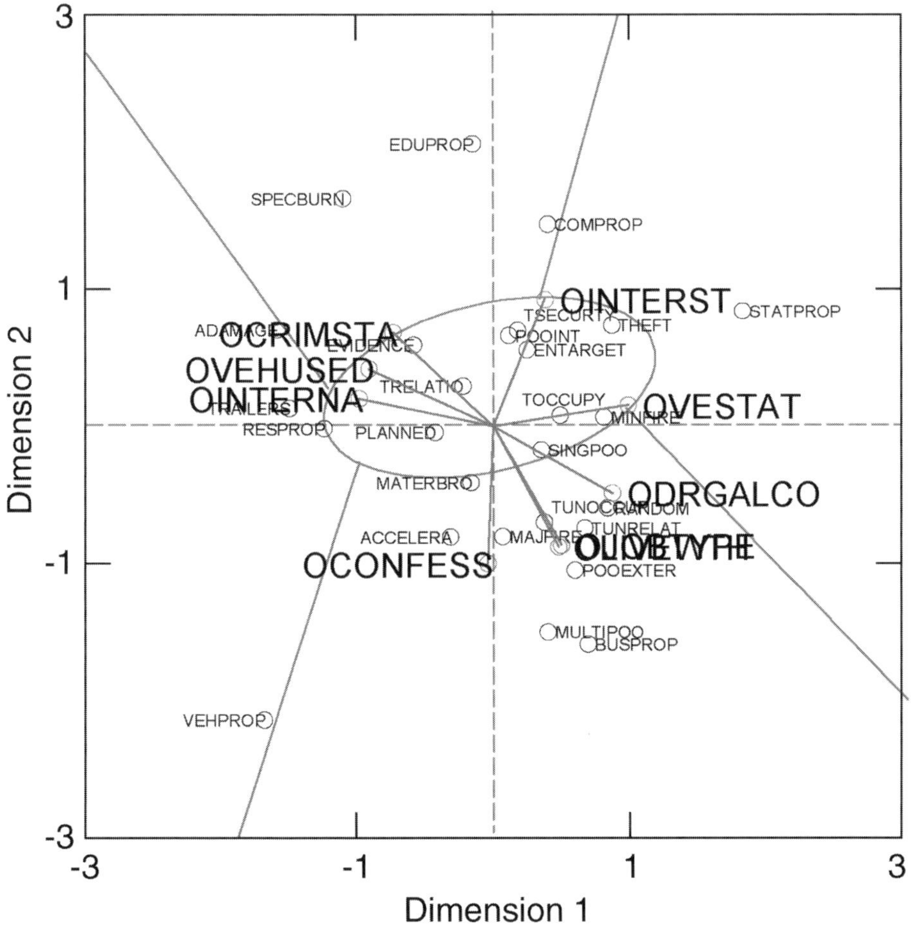

Fig. 9.3. Fitted (significant) general offender behavior pattern vectors.

be most useful in profiling serial arsonists. It should be noted that certain crime scene variables may be missing from a specific figure because of the presence of missing observations for that particular variable in the property-fitting analysis. Where this occurs, the reader will note slight but inconsequential perturbations in the preference mapping scaling solution represented. In Appendix G, Table 1 provides relevant numerical data (e.g., standardized regression weights, multiple *r* values, omnibus *F*-test values, and *p* values) used to facilitate the property-fitting exercise for the personal, general, and event-specific variable sets, respectively. Table 1 in Appendix G also lists

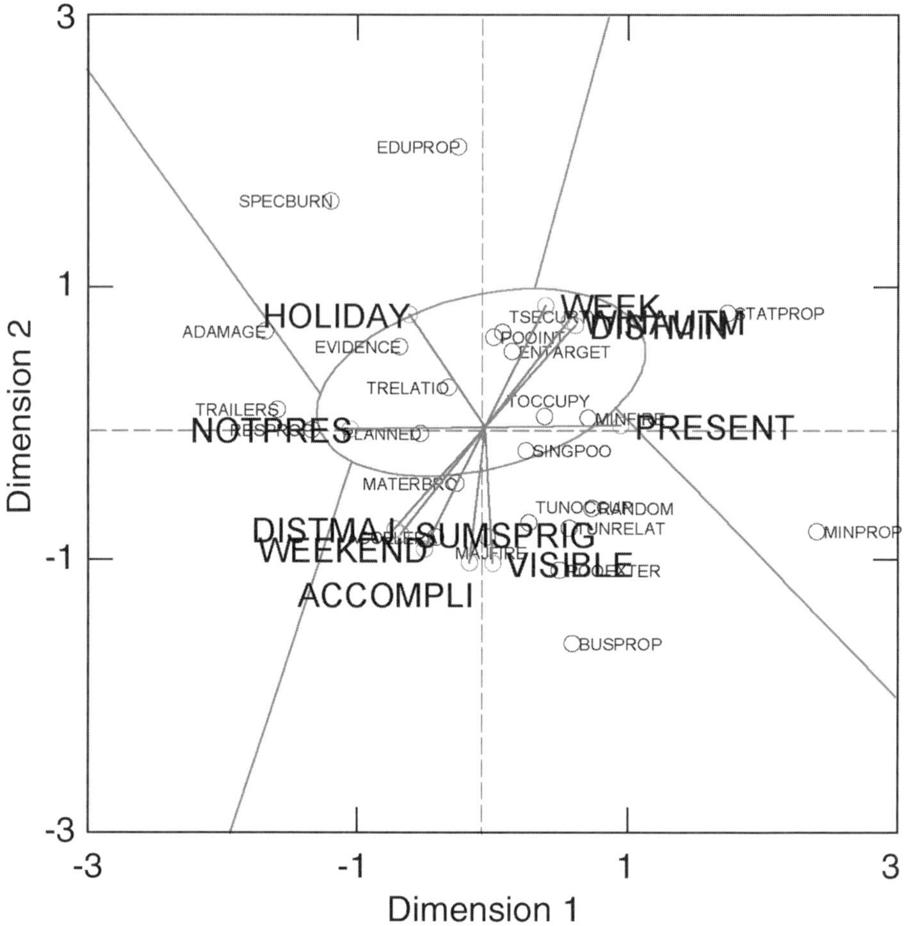

Fig. 9.4. Fitted (significant) event-specific offender behavior and choice pattern vectors.

those external property variables whose fitted vectors are not displayed in the figures by virtue of not being significantly predicted by the two-dimensional MDS coordinates. These variables are therefore largely irrelevant for achieving an understanding of the association between crime scene variables and offender-related variables.

Interpretation of Figs. 9.2 through 9.4, one plot for each of the three conceptual sets of offender-related external variables, is relatively straightforward, especially when interpreted in conjunction with the regions identified in Fig. 9.1 and the interpretations of the dimensions offered in the previous section. Each fitted vector on a figure summarizes the relationship that exists between a specific external offender-related variable and the two dimensions (i.e., the spatial pattern) of the MDS solution. The strength of the relationship is measured by the multiple correlation between the two dimensional coordinates and the conditional probability scores for the variables. The direction of the relationship directly reflects the combination of signs of the standardized regression weights for the two dimensions. Therefore, movement toward the circle along a particular vector is interpreted as reflecting an increasing tendency (i.e., the conditional probability that the offender-related variable takes on a value of 1 when a crime scene variable takes on a value of 1) for the offender-related variable to take on a coded value of 1 in association with the crime scene variables in the region of the circle and vice versa when moving in the opposite direction.

Personal Offender Characteristics

Figure. 9.2 shows fitted property vectors for six significant personal characteristics of offenders. The offender language (OLANG) and offender accent (OACCENT) vectors showed higher conditional probabilities with crime scene characteristics falling toward the planning/deliberation end of dimension 1, especially oriented toward the cluster 3 region. Thus, there were higher probabilities that the offender was at least bilingual and spoke with an accent at crime scenes in which the TRAILERS, RESPROP, and VEHPROP variables took on a coded value of 1. The offender hair and eye color vectors (OHAIRCOL and OEYECOL) generally suggested a higher probability of offenders having darker hair and eyes and involving crime scenes targeting commercial and state-owned properties where sexual activity was evident (cluster 5 orientation). The offender teeth and features vectors (OTEETH and OUTFEAT) revealed higher probabilities of offenders having noticeably imperfect teeth and an outstanding feature, respectively, at the more random outdoor crime scenes that had multiple points of entry and were unrelated to the offender (cluster 2 orientation). Finally, readers are reminded that the data originate from police records. Consequently, some of the offenders' personal characteristic variables were included to provide descriptive richness to the results. These results should not be interpreted or used in any manner that would suggest racial stereotyping.

General Offender Behavior Variables

Figure 9.3 shows the fitted property vectors for nine significant general offender behaviors. The offender criminal status, vehicle, and international vectors (OCRIMSTAT, OVEHUSED, and OINTERNA) generally suggested higher probabilities of offenders having a prior criminal status, using a vehicle to commit crimes, and having been overseas within the past 10 years at crime scenes especially associated with clusters 2 and 4 and the small subregion of cluster 1 (using trailers, targeting educational and residential properties, causing other damage to targets, starting fires with specific items, and leaving evidence). The offender interstate vector (OINTERST) revealed a higher probability of offenders having traveled out of state within the past 10 years at crime scenes oriented toward clusters 4 and 5 and the outer fringes of cluster 1 (targeting especially educational, commercial and state-owned properties where theft tends to also occur), and having facial hair and darker hair color and shade. The offender vehicle status vector (OVESTAT) showed a higher probability of offenders not owning the vehicle used in a crime at crime scenes especially associated with cluster 5 and the outer fringes of cluster 1 (where state-owned properties are targeted, theft tends to occur, and minor fires result). The offender drug and alcohol, cohabitation, and job type vectors (ODRGALCO, OLIVEWTH, and OJOBTYPE) suggested higher probabilities of offenders showing evidence of drug or alcohol use, living with other people, and being employed at crime scenes especially associated with cluster 2 variables (random acts at targets unrelated to the offender, targeting bush properties, with points of origin exterior to the target). The offender confession vector (OCONFESS) suggested a higher probability of offenders having confessed to similar crimes at crime scenes especially associated with the more deliberative subregion of cluster 2 (where accelerants are used, a major fire results, and materials are brought to the target by the offender).

Event-Specific Offender Behaviors and Choices Variables

Figure 9.4 shows the fitted property vectors for 11 significant event-specific offender behaviors and choices. It should be noted that some of these vectors are concerned with the offender's choice of timing for the arson crime and the remainder concern actions of the offender taken in relation to a specific arson event. The time-related vectors will be interpreted first. The HOLIDAY vector suggested a higher probability of the offender committing a crime of arson during holiday periods, at crime scenes associated particularly with cluster 4 and the small subregion of cluster 1 (where educational properties are targeted, specific items are used to start the fire, evidence is left behind, the offender is related to the target, and other damage is done to the target). This relationship pattern is probably most closely linked to vandalism activity at schools during holiday periods. The WEEK vector was more oriented toward both cluster 4 and 5 variables and the outer fringes of cluster 1. Here, a higher probability of offenders choosing weekdays for their crimes was associated with crime scenes showing features such as educational or state-owned properties, where security systems were present, theft was likely to have occurred, point of origin of the fire was interior to the target, and there was evidence that the offender actually entered the target. The WEEKEND vector showed the opposite directional trend in which offenders tended to choose a weekend day to start their fires and this was associated with those crime scene variables located in the more planned subregion of cluster 2 (where materials were brought to the target, accelerants were used, and a major fire resulted). The summer–spring and winter–autumn vectors (SUMSPRIG and WINAUTM) tended to work almost in parallel (i.e, showing nearly identical association patterns) with the WEEKEND and WEEK vectors, respectively.

With respect to event-specific offender behaviors, the PRESENT vector suggested a higher probability of the offender actually being present at the crime scene during the fire, at crime scenes associated with cluster 5 (where the crime was random rather than planned, state-owned property or minor property had been targeted, small fires resulted, and theft was likely to have occurred). The not present vector (NOTPRES) worked in the opposite direction, suggesting that offenders tended not to be present at crimes that had been planned and accelerants and trailers had been used. The accomplice and visible vectors (ACCOMPLI and VISIBLE) were nearly parallel and revealed higher probabilities of offenders working with accomplices and starting their fires in a visible area with possible witnesses, at crime scenes associated strongly with cluster 2 features (where targets tended to be outdoors with multiple and exterior points of origin for fires, targets were unoccupied, the crime tended to be random rather than planned, and a major fire ensued).

Conclusion

The results discussed in this chapter have yielded an empirical model for serial arson crime scene behaviors (depicted in Fig. 9.1) that can be systematically associated with probable offender characteristics (Figs. 9.2–9.4). The model depicted in Fig. 9.1 shows that serial arson crime scene behaviors are composed of a centrally located constellation of common behaviors surrounded by four outlying patterns. Each of these outlying patterns represents a distinct and coherent style in the commission of a serial arson attack.

Focusing first on the central cluster, it can be seen that serial arson is composed of a broad constellation of common behaviors which also contain a further subset of behaviors (shown by the smaller, dotted ellipse), more closely related to crime scene behaviors to the left of Fig. 9.1. These common behaviors provide a core description of the characteristic behaviors common to all patterns of serial arson. The subset indicates that crime patterns toward the left of Fig. 9.1 are quite likely to contain these three specific behaviors. Thus, for example, cluster 3 will have a very high propensity for planning in the commission of the offense, a relationship between the victim and target, and evidence to be left at the crime scene.

A number of interesting theoretical implications emerge when considering the significance of the behaviors located in the common behavior cluster. The common presence of planning and evidence in the commission of most offenses is at odds with the basic tenet of the organized–disorganized behavior dichotomy. The main premise of the dichotomy is the categorical distinction of behaviors by their offense sophistication. The presence of planning is suggestive of an organized offender with its absence indicative of a disorganized offender. However, given that planning is located in the common behavior cluster indicates that generally all serial arson offenses will typically involve this, which therefore questions the validity of such a categorical distinction. Similarly, the common presence of evidence at most serial arson crime scenes is not congruent with the concept of the organized–disorganized dichotomy, which cites the detection of evidence as a key indicator of a disorganized offender (*17*, p. 166).

This incidence of planning as a central element to all serial arson offenses is matched by the observation that some form of relationship usually exists between the victim and offender. This result is contrary to previous conceptions describing these crimes as seemingly random and motiveless *(29)* and suggests that on some psychological level there is indeed coherency or, proverbially speaking, a method to their madness. Examples of this relationship can range from cognitive knowledge of their environment to some internal fantasy that is then superimposed on the presented target. From an investigative perspective, this aspect may prove especially useful because it suggests that careful consideration of the target may provide insight into an offender. Indeed, the nature of this relation may especially become more overt when considered in conjunction with behaviors derived in one of the outlying patterns.

This theme of planning as a central element of all such offenses is congruent with those observed in the previous two chapters concerned with the study of sexual murder and serial rapes. Indeed, these findings support those of Kocsis et al. *(18)* in highlighting the theoretical limitations of the organized–disorganized dichotomy and the limitations of such a categorical classification.

In looking at the other actions encompassed by the common behaviors cluster, a number of other features emerge concerning the inherent nature of serial arson crimes. Provided the target is a structure, arsonists commonly enter their target, steal items if available, and then initiate small fires with single internal points of origin. This is particularly interesting because offenders may engage in such behaviors even though the target may be equipped with various security and–or fire retardant devices or even occupied by individuals who may detect and apprehend them. This constellation of behaviors suggests that the inherent psychological nature of serial arson is a somewhat brazen crime that does not concord with common behavior patterns observable in other crime modalities, such as murder or rape, in which offenders are typically deterred by a greater degree of risk of apprehension or a diminished capacity to complete their crime.

Turning to the first of the outlying behavior patterns, the *thrill* pattern (cluster 2) is the only outlying pattern containing a subset of behaviors differentiated along dimension 1 (i.e., from left to right) of Fig. 9.1. The *thrill* pattern embodies a somewhat sporadic style of offense. However, this sporadic nature should not be mistaken for incoherence as in the disorganized offender category, but rather, is suggestive of multiple targets being attacked. This nuance is more apparent when it is recognized that the *thrill* pattern can nonetheless demonstrate quite sophisticated and premeditated behaviors.

Indeed, the distinguishing element between the subsets of the *thrill* pattern is evidence of behavioral sophistication, such as the use of various resources to initiate a fire. Thus, the subset to the left is represented by behaviors such as the offender using materials and accelerants that subsequently result in a much larger fire. The subset to the right is characterized more by behaviors concerned with committing multiple attacks on comparatively unrelated targets. Greater insight into the nature of any offender's target relationship is more apparent when one considers that the predominant target in this pattern is some form of bush, forest, or vegetation. The scope of possible relationships between such targets is lessened in comparison with other targets, such as, for example, a residence with which the offender harbors a prior grievance with the occupant.

A curious set of offender characteristics emerge as being associated with this style of offense. In physical appearance, these offenders tend to have poor dental work and some type of outstanding physical feature (e.g., scarring). Additionally, this pattern will typically be comprised of multiple offenders who are employed, live with others (i.e., they are not social loners), and ingest alcohol and/or drugs before the commission of an offense. Because they commonly travel more than 1 mile to commit an offense, they will typically be quite mobile. Looking at temporal features, these offenders usually commit their offenses in summer–spring months and predominantly on weekends. Finally, offenders are characterized by other factors. First, they will initiate a fire in a highly visible location where they may be potentially identified and apprehended. Second, these offenders are likely to confess to having committed other similar crimes after apprehension.

What emerges from this pattern are older individuals who are socially competent in their lives, cognitively aware of their actions, and yet engage in a high degree of risk to commit offenses of arson (hence the *thrill* label for this pattern). Unlike the other patterns discussed herein, no significant element of animosity appears to exist with this pattern. Instead, these offenders seem to derive satisfaction from the destruction of property. Although they are not explicitly sexual in their behaviors, the fact that these offenders are typically older and physically unattractive may suggest the sublimation of a possible sexual drive. Thus, this pattern holds some similarities to the broad excitement category proposed by Douglas et al. *(17)*. This pattern seems to encapsulate a theme of recreational fascination with fire. Some anecdotal case examples of this psychological pattern include firefighters seeking to create some activity for themselves or bored teenagers deriving excitement from the risk of starting a fire. These scenario-based examples are quite different but both share the underlying theme of the *thrill* pattern in creating excitement or entertainment for the perpetrator through fire setting.

The next outlying behavior pattern (cluster 3), labeled the *anger* pattern, involves a style of offense in which some form of animosity or rage seems to find expression in the commission of an arson attack. A significant feature of this behavior pattern is that targets are predominantly residential properties or motor vehicles. This distinction in target selection is important because it suggests that the violence in the crime is associated with expressing or inflicting personalized harm rather than general destruction inflicted on some conceptual organization or entity. Indeed, this intent to cause harm also finds expression in the other two characteristic behaviors in this pattern. First, offenders employ trailers to ensure the thorough spread of the fire. Of more significance, however, is that the offender's anger will typically find further expression in physically destroying household items in addition to the subsequent damage caused by igniting a fire. So, for example, an offender will enter the residence and then manually destroy some of the household items (e.g., television, stereo system) before commencing a fire.

The perpetrators of such crimes in the current sample tend to be foreign nationals who are bilingual and consequently tend to possess a noticeable accent. They also hold a certain degree of financial stability because they possess and use a vehicle for transport. Finally, burning the target does not appear to hold any deeper psychological meaning other than to inflict harm; consequently, they typically decamp from the crime scene once the fire has been lit.

At a cursory level, there are similarities between the *anger* pattern and previously developed conceptions, such as the revenge-motivated arsonist described by Douglas et al. *(17)* or the instrumental person proposed by Canter and Fritzon *(21)*. However, a number of important differences exist between these previous conceptions and the *anger* pattern. Foremost is the nature of the relationship between the offender and the target. Both the revenge motive and the instrumental person pattern share the identical theme of retaliation and retribution as underlying the expressed actions of the offense. However, the concept of a prior relationship between the target and the offender in the present study is based more on cognitive knowledge or recognition of the target. Consequently, an offender in the *anger* pattern may not actually harbor any previous animosity toward or grievance with the target, but may instead attack because of some perceived familiarity or recognition. This distinction is further highlighted because the *anger* pattern describes the actions of serial arsonists, whereas the revenge motive and instrumental person are both primarily conceived as relating to a non-recidivistic offense that finds expression in a very specific target. Indeed, the theme of the *anger* pattern is similar to that found in the studies discussed in the previous two chapters examining sexual murderers and serial rapists. Both types of offenders exhibit a behavior pattern involving the expression of an unfocused internal rage on a target.

Cluster 4 has been labeled as the *resentment* pattern. The theme of this pattern appears to be a generalized sentiment of animosity visited on a vague class of target. Thus, the *resentment* pattern predominantly features attacks on churches or educational facilities, such as schools and universities, or on commercial properties, such as business establishments. Additionally, offenders in this pattern will initially ignite specific items within the target; the destruction of these items first is suggestive of some specific meaning to the offender. Offenders associated with this pattern typically possess a prior criminal history and frequently perpetrate their attacks on weekends.

There is some similarity between the theme of the *resentment* pattern and previous categorizations, such as vandalism-motivated arson *(17)* or the instrumental object offense pattern described by Canter and Fritzon *(21)*. These similarities primarily exist because of the unfocused nature of the attacks. However, akin to the observations in the *anger* pattern, these previous categorizations were not specifically developed in considering the actions of a serial offender. When focusing exclusively on targeting educational facilities, some resemblance exists between the resentment pattern and a crime phenomenon referred to as school fires *(30)* in which educational facilities are specifically attacked by juveniles. This specific scenario also suggests that these offenses occur predominately on weekends. Nonetheless, these previous conceptions fail to adequately explain the potential existence of an element of animosity as expressed by the initial burning of specific items or the propensity for commercial properties to also be attacked in similar circumstances. Clearly, this pattern warrants further scrutiny in any future research.

The fifth and final cluster is labeled the *sexual* pattern and embodies an offense style in which the offender associates the ignition of fires with sexual excitement and/or gratification. The most distinguishing behavioral element of this pattern is evidence of sexual activity by the offender at or near the crime scene. The common targets in this offense pattern are state-owned (public), easily accessible premises, such as trash receptacles, post boxes, public toilets, or any other publicly accessible facility. These arson attacks are relatively minor in size and do not typically escalate into major fires that cause serious destruction. Indeed, this pattern demonstrates the lowest amount of behavioral sophistication and as such the regional interpretation of the data is found in the far right of Fig. 9.1.

Looking at typical offender characteristics associated with this pattern, offenders are likely to have dark-colored hair and eyes and a history of domestic travel, however, not by their own vehicle. In the commission of their offenses these offenders do not generally travel far and typically light fires on weekdays and during winter and/or autumn months. However, of most significance with this behavioral pattern is that these offenders have a tendency to remain at the crime scene to typically observe the fire and/or its extinguishment.

The *sexual* pattern holds a number of clear similarities to previous psychiatric/psychological studies of arsonists in the context of representing a form of sexual perversion or paraphilic compulsion that has been made with fire setting *(4,7)*. However, within the context of profiling literature the sexual pattern has a number of similarities to the excitement motive described by Douglas et al. *(17)* or the expressive object offense pattern observed by Canter and Fritzon *(21)*. Indeed, the expressive object pattern is described as the only arson behavior pattern being recidivistic in nature in terms of involving the selection of public buildings as common targets, and being connected with the achievement of some form of emotional relief. Despite these similarities, a number of notable inconsistencies are also apparent. Although the expressive object pattern is said to be instigated to achieve some emotional relief, the exact nature of the relief is not typically explicit and consequently may not equate with sexual perversion. Additionally, the selected targets described in the expressive object conveys the impression of large structures being targeted (e.g., hospitals, businesses), whereas the typical victim class in the *sexual* pattern is more in the nature of minor nuisance fires on small, public, and easily accessed targets.

In conclusion, the present results offer an empirical model against which serial arson behaviors can systematically be assessed. The key feature of this model is the holistic depiction of all potential behavioral patterns, both common and discriminatory, that are not inherently formulated on the inference of potential motives. This empirically based model serves as a practical tool for the practice of profiling in the context of a serial arson crime series because behaviors can be assessed using the model to provide insight into both the style of the offense and the offender's unique personal characteristics.

ACKNOWLEDGMENT

This chapter is sourced from material previously published by Kocsis, R. N. and Cooksey, R. W. (2002). Criminal psychological profiling of serial arson crimes. Int J Offender Ther Comp Criminol, 46(4), 631–656.

REFERENCES

1. Holmes, R.M. and Holmes, S.T. (1996). Profiling violent crimes: An investigative tool, 2nd ed. Thousand Oaks, CA: Sage.
2. Rossmo, D.K. (1997). Geographic profiling. In: Jackson, J.L. and Berkerian, D.A., eds. Offender profiling: Theory, research and practice. New York: Wiley, pp.159–175.
3. Vorpagel, R.E. (1982). Painting psychological profiles: Charlatanism, coincidence, charisma or new science. Police Chief, 3(8), 156–159.
4. Barnett, W. and Spitzer, M. (1994). Pathological fire-setting 1951–1991: A review. Medicine, Science, and Law, 34(1), 4–20.
5. Geller, J.L. (1992). Pathological firesetting in adults. International Journal of Law Psychiatry, 15, 283–302.
6. Harris, G.T. and Rice, M.E. (1996). A typology of mentally disordered firesetters. Journal of Interpersonal Violence, 22, 351–363.
7. Lewis, N.D.C. and Yarnell, H. (1952). Pathological fire-setting (pyromania) (nervous and mental disease monograph, no. 82). New York: Coolidge Foundation.
8. Rix, K.J.B. (1994). A psychiatric study of adult arsonists. Medicine, Science, and Law, 34(1), 21–34.
9. Bennett, W.M. and Hess, K.M. (1984). The arsonist: A closer look. Investigating arson. Springfield, IL: Thomas.
10. Prins, H., Tennent, G., Trick, K. (1985). Motives for arson (fire raising). Medicine, Science, and Law, 25(4), 275–278.
11. Orr, J. (1989). Profiles in arson: The serial firesetter. American Fire Journal, 32, 24–27, 32, 33.
12. Orr, J. (1989). Profiles in arson: The revenge firesetter. American Fire Journal, 33, 30–32.
13. Jeffers, H.P. (1992). Profiles in evil. London: Warner Bros.
14. Icove, D. J. and Estepp, M. H. (1987). Motive-based offender profiles of arson and fire-related crimes. FBI Law Enforcement Bulletin, 56(4), 17–23.

15. Rider, A.O. (1980). The firesetter: A psychological profile. Part 1. FBI Law Enforcement Bulletin, 49(6), 6–13.
16. Rider, A.O. (1980). The firesetter: A psychological profile. Part 2. FBI Law Enforcement Bulletin, 49(7), 12–17.
17. Douglas, J.E., Burgess, A.W., Burgess, A.G., Ressler, R.K. (1992). Crime classification manual. London: Simon & Schuster.
18. Kocsis, R.N., Irwin, H.J., Hayes, A. F. (1998). Organised and disorganised behavior syndromes in arsonists: A validation study of a psychological profiling concept. Psychiatry, Psychology and Law, 5, 117–130.
19. Ressler, R.K., Burgess, A.W., Douglas, J.E. (1988). Sexual homicide: Patterns and motives. New York: Lexington Books.
20. Canter, D. and Heritage, R. (1989). A multivariate model of sexual offence behaviour: Developments in offender profiling. International Journal of Forensic Psychiatry, 1, 185–212.
21. Canter, D. and Fritzon, K. (1998). Differentiating arsonists: A model of firesetting actions and characteristics. Legal and Criminological Psychology, 3, 73–96.
22. Geberth, V.J. (1996). Practical homicide investigation, 2nd ed. New York: CRC Press.
23. Britton, P. (1997). The jigsaw man. London: Bantam Press.
24. Dietz, P.E. (1985). Sex offender profiling by the FBI: A preliminary conceptual model. In: Ben-Aron, M.H., Hucher, S.J., Webster, C.D., eds. Clinical Criminology. Toronto: M & M Graphics, pp. 207–219.
25. Douglas, J.E., Ressler, R.K., Burgess, A.W., Hartman, C.R. (1986). Criminal profiling from crime scene analysis. Behavioral Science and Law, 4, 401–421.
26. Hair, J.F. Jr., Anderson, R.E., Tatham, R.L., Black, W.G. (1998). Multivariate data analysis, 5th ed. Upper Saddle River, NJ: Prentice Hall.
27. Coxon, A.P.M. (1982). The user's guide to multidimensional scaling. London: Heinemann Educational Books.
28. Kruskal, J.B. and Wish, M. (1978). Multidimensional scaling. Beverly Hills, CA: Sage.
29. Holmes, R.M. and Holmes, S.T. (1998). Serial murder, 2nd ed. Newbury Park, CA: Sage.
30. Burns, L. (1991). School arson in New South Wales. Sydney: Government Printer.

Chapter 10

Offense Location Patterns

Geographic Profiles

Summary

In addition to describing the biographical features of an unknown offender, criminal profiles can also provide some indication of the general area where an offender may be found to reside and/or hold some type of relationship based on the spatial locations of the committed offenses. This chapter discusses CAP research within this area and then describes a series of systematic steps whereby such spatial patterns can be assessed to develop what is now commonly referred to as a geographic profile.

Key Words: Spatial offense locations; geographic profiles.

Introduction

Virtually any contemporary criminal investigation involves finding the answer to two fundamental questions: who committed the crime and where can they be found? The first involves determining the identity of the perpetrator(s) of a crime and the second involves establishing where the criminal(s) may be apprehended. Previous chapters of this book discussed various studies that offered models that could be used to generate predictions of descriptive characteristics of an offender, such as age, gender, and marital status. Consequently, these chapters serve to address the first question relating to the identity of the offender. However, in addressing the question of where the perpetrator may be apprehended, a subcategory of criminal profiling has evolved that is now commonly referred to as geographic profiling.

The theoretical basis of geographic profiling centers around the notion that most criminal offenders do not travel far from their residence when com-

From: *Criminal Profiling: Principles and Practice*
By: R. N. Kocsis © Humana Press Inc., Totowa, NJ

mitting a crime. Throughout this chapter the term *residence* will be used as a shorthand expression to describe a location that has some geographical nexus or connection with an offender, serving as a point of orientation for his or her movement patterns. Thus, an offender may choose to commit offenses in areas located, for example, close to their area of residence, work, recreational activity, or where they own a property. Consequently, a geographic profile attempts to make a prediction concerning an offender's likely place of orientation that is intrinsically connected to him or her based on the spatial locations of offenses. This is typically accomplished by plotting offense locations on some type of map and using various measurements to identify an area most likely to have some significance to the offender. Consequently, it is important to appreciate that geographic profiling differs from the bulk of criminological literature concerned with the geographic analysis of offense locations, which has tended to focus on offense locations on a much larger scale such as, for example, offense distributions across wider demographics such as whole cities *(1–3)*.

Contrary to some promulgated views, the concept of identifying an offender's whereabouts based on the location of his or her offenses is neither a recent nor revolutionary concept. Indeed, investigators have engaged in the construction of various types of pin maps to gain some insight into an offense series for numerous decades *(4–6)*. Arguably, however, what has transpired in recent years, especially within the field of criminal profiling, has been a major invigoration of interest in the concept. The basis for this resurgence of interest appears to be related to the availability of now reasonably affordable computer programs known as geographic information systems (GIS), which allow for the quick and comparatively easy construction of maps for a wide range of applications and purposes. In this context, a large proportion of contemporary research in the area of geographic profiling predominantly focuses on the development of a geographic profile by the use of a computer system. This has led in turn to a proliferation of commercial computer products that can generate geographic profiles from a set of crime locations that have been input into a computer software program *(7–9)*.

Although these programs generate impressive graphical displays via the presentation of maps depicting a geographic profile, they are not without their limitations. With the focus on the development of geographic profiling techniques reliant on such computer applications, the constituent principles and measurements underpinning these programs is often increasingly difficult to scrutinize or verify. In many circumstances, the development of a geographic profile is dependent on accessing appropriate computer hardware in conjunction with a given geographic profiling program.

Another difficulty associated with computerized geographic profiling systems relates to their utility. Although these programs are visually impressive in terms of pictorial representations and maps they are capable of producing, the information generated by these programs may not in practice surpass what can be accomplished by more rudimentary forms of measurement and maps *(10)*. This issue was explored in a study by Snook et al. *(11)* that compared the predictions of a group of students given some rudimentary training in geographic profiling with the predictions generated by a computerized geographic profiling program. The results of this study found little difference in the achieved results between the computerized system and the techniques employed by the students.

In recognition of the burgeoning popularity of geographic profiling research, however, the author set about identifying a series of user-friendly principles and geometric measurements that could be applied for the generation of a geographic profile without the need for any sophisticated computer system.

The Fundamentals of Geographic Profiling

Before explaining how a geographic profile can be generated, some understanding of the principles underpinning the various geometric measurements is required. In this regard, many of the principles developed for the construction of a geographic profile articulated herein represent developments of principles first articulated by Canter and Larkin *(12)*. In attempting to develop some system whereby offense locations could be systematically evaluated and used to generate some impression of an offender's likely residence, a number of theoretical assumptions were made by Canter and Larkin *(12)*, the most fundamental of which being that any system seeking to predict an offender's place of residence assumes that the offender in question operates from some established place of residence or base. Consequently, all of the principles discussed herein are unlikely to work in the circumstance of an itinerant offender who lacks any fixed place of abode.

The next theoretical assumption involved consideration of how the human mind operates to orientate an individual through their environment when traveling to commit a crime. In addressing this issue, two theoretical constructs were proposed. The first was the *home range* that effectively represents an individual's total spatial knowledge of their environment that also encompasses their place of residence. The second was the *criminal range* that represents the conceptual area wherein an individual is prepared to travel to commit their crime(s). Accordingly, the principles of geographic profiling essentially require the reconciliation of the mental processes operating in an offender's mind when traveling between the two ranges; that is, the home and the criminal range to commit a crime.

Based on previous criminological research examining the geographic distributions of offenses, Canter and Larkin *(12)* reasoned that the relationship between the conceptual home and criminal ranges would not be purely random. Consequently, they proposed two hypothetical models respectively entitled *commuter* and *marauder*. The commuter model proposes a movement pattern in which an offender moves from his or her residence to a location to commit offenses that are not necessarily limited by the parameters of their conceptual home range. The central idea behind the commuter model is that little or no overlap exists between an offender's conceptual criminal range and his or her home range that typically encapsulates their residence. Consequently, the commuter model describes a circumstance whereby an offender can potentially travel to an area far beyond the boundaries of his or her conceptual home range to commit a crime.

In many respects, the marauder model is the opposite of the commuter model. The marauder model describes a movement pattern wherein the offender's place of residence acts as a central point of orientation from which he or she may move out in all directions to commit offenses and then return to his or her home or base. This style of movement in committing crimes is referred to as a domocentric movement pattern and is illustrated in Fig. 10.1.

An important feature of the marauder model is that it ascribes a strong relationship between the criminal and home ranges that contains the offender's residence. Consequently, in the marauder model, the home and criminal ranges overlap one another and the criminal range is typically constrained by the boundaries of the home range. Thus, in the circumstance of the marauder model, an offender will not travel beyond the boundaries of his or her home range to commit an offense in an area that is unfamiliar to him or her. Having made these conceptual assumptions, a method was needed to test their validity. The first step in this process involved developing a method to measure the conceptual criminal range. This was accomplished by first plotting a series of offenses on a map. Once all offense locations were plotted the distance between the two furthest offenses was used as the diameter to draw and identify a circle on the map. It was reasoned that if this technique of plotting a circle was an adequate measure of the conceptual criminal range then the circle should encapsulate most, if not all, of the plotted offense locations. With the development of this circle measurement as a representation of the conceptual criminal range, the next step then involved considering its relationship with the location of an offender's residence. The assumption underpinning the commuter model is that offenders can travel to an area beyond the boundaries of their

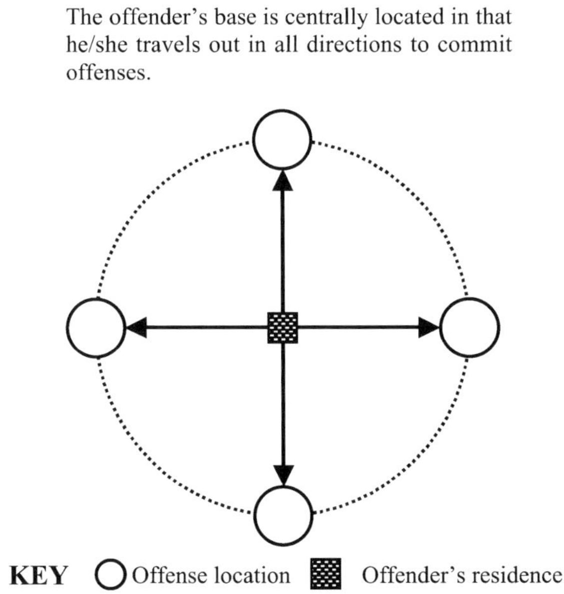

Fig. 10.1. The domocentric movement pattern encapsulates the principles of the marauder model, whereby an offender's residence is positioned within an area framed by the location of the offenses.

home range that encapsulates their place of residence. Consequently, in the circumstance of the commuter model, an offender's residence would not necessarily be found within the boundary of the circle measurement used as an estimation of the criminal range. However, in direct contrast, the principles of the marauder model suggest a strong overlap between the home and criminal ranges. If an offender were behaving in accordance with the principles of the marauder model and the offense locations plotted on a map with the circle measurement drawn between the two furthest offenses, then the offender's residence, in this circumstance, would be likely to be located somewhere within the boundaries of the circle.

These propositions were tested by obtaining the offense locations and home locations of 45 cases of serial rape. With this information, the offense and offender's home locations from each of the 45 cases were plotted on a separate map and a diametric circle between the two furthest offense locations drawn on each of the maps. Following this procedure it was found that the circle measurement encapsulated all of the offense locations in 91% of the cases. Consequently, this indicated that the circle measurement was a reasonably reliable measure of the conceptual criminal range. The next step then was

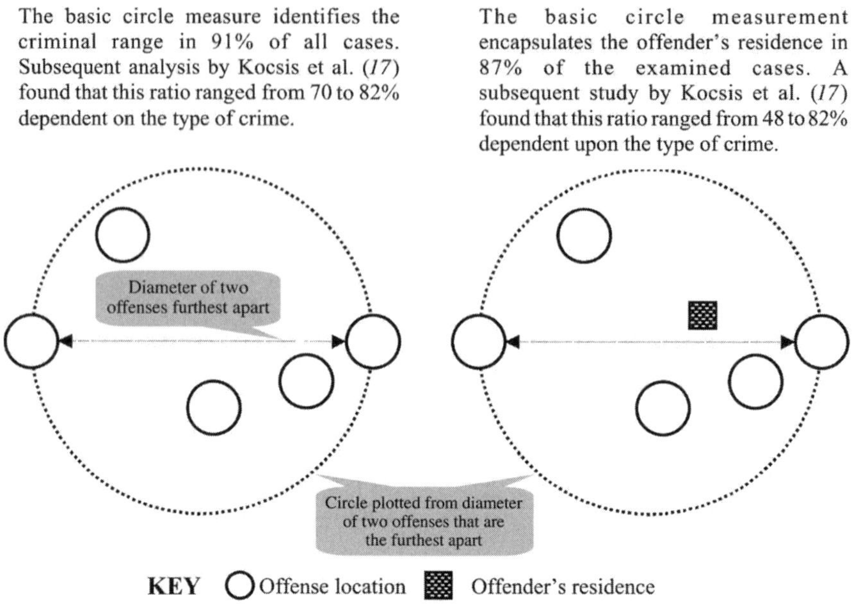

Fig. 10.2. Hypothetical examples of offense patterns that conform to the principles of the basic circle measurement and the domocentric movement pattern that encapsulates the offender's probable area of residence.

to observe the location of the offender's residence relative to the drawn circle in each of the 45 maps. When the respective locations of each offender's residence were examined it was found to be within the boundaries of the circle in 87% of the cases. Figure 10.2 illustrates these findings using the basic circle measurement.

With these findings, the basis for a method of predicting an offender's area of residence (i.e., a geographic profile) can be developed by reversing the principles. First, this involves plotting the locations of a series of offenses on a map. Second, a line that can be drawn between the two offenses that are the furthest apart forms the diameter of a circle. Relying on the findings of Canter and Larkin *(12)*, this circle is likely to have a high (i.e., 91%) probability of depicting the offender's area of criminal activity as well as possessing a good chance (i.e., 87%) of encompassing the location of the offender's residence.

Developing the Circle Measurement for Practical Application

The concepts involved in the circle measurement appear relatively straightforward in that by following the steps predictions can be made concerning an offender's likely area of residence. However, applying these principles in the context of an actual criminal investigation is somewhat more problematic. For example, the circle measurement prescribes the plotting of a diametric circle from the two furthest offenses. The space within this circle will feasibly have a high probability of encompassing the location of the offender's residence. However, given the diversity of serial offenders *(13–15)*, a number of questions arise in applying this measurement. For example, will this technique work effectively across any type of serial crime or only in the circumstance of serial rapists? Also, when can the circle measurement be effectively applied in the circumstance of an on-going sequence of offenses? Namely, can it be applied after the commission of merely two offenses or are more required to effectively assess the offender's movement pattern? The principles of the circle measurement were developed in an experiment that used the locations of all offenses in retrospect when the offender had already been apprehended and all offense locations identified. Finally, although the basic circle measurement proposes a method for predicting an area likely to contain the offender's residence, is the size of this area practically useful? Hypothetically speaking, a system could be developed that could always be arguably correct by the identification of a gigantic prediction area. Rather than predicting an area so large as to be of no practical value, however, are there any techniques of measurement that could potentially reduce and thus focus the prediction area into one of more practical utility?

Although Canter and Larkin *(12)* initially proposed the principle of circle measurement in comparatively simple terms, their subsequent endeavors have apparently become increasingly oriented toward developing geographic profiling within the context of a computerized system *(16)*. As previously mentioned, this development promotes the necessity of using a computer program often with little or no opportunity to scrutinize the tenets of its construction. It was with this in mind then that the CAP research was undertaken to try and develop a systemized method for developing a geographic profile that did not require the use of any computerized system. Instead, principles were developed to allow for the development of a geographic profile by manually plotting an easy geometric measurement on a map.

Crime Modality

Possibly the most fundamental question concerning the circle measurement is in what circumstance can it be applied? Are these principles applicable to all forms of serial crime or only serial rapists? Given the varying factors motivating different types of crime, there is quite justifiable reason to question the applicability of the circle measurement to various types of crime. Two CAP studies thus far have considered this question. The first by Kocsis and Irwin *(17)* tested the basic principles of the circle measurement with samples of serial rapists, arsonists, and burglars. This study concluded that the basic circle measurement encompassed all offenses, and thus provided a depiction of the conceptual criminal range, in 79% of the serial rape cases, 82% of the serial arson cases, and 70% of the serial (i.e., repeat) burglary cases studied. However, with respect to where the offender's residence was located relative to the boundaries of the circle it was found that the circle encompassed the respective offender's home in 71% of the serial rape cases, 82% of the serial arson cases, and only 48% of the burglary cases. In a subsequent study, Kocsis et al. *(18)* again tested the applicability of the basic circle measurement in the context of serial burglary. The results of this study were consistent with its predecessor with the circle measurement encapsulating an offender's residence in exactly half (50%) of the tested cases.

The results of these studies suggest a number of things. First, they indicate that the principles of the circle measurement may not be as effective as perhaps first thought and initially proposed by Canter and Larkin *(12)*. That is, the frequency of the circle measurement encompassing all offenses and thus acting as a conceptual representation of the area of criminal activity ranged from 70 to 82% reliability across the differing sampled crime modalities, whereas the frequency of the circle measurement encompassing the offender's residence ranged between 48 and 82%. Although these results are supportive, they do not appear as optimistic as Canter and Larkin's *(12)* results. It would also seem that the principles of the circle measurement are not as likely to be effective in accounting for the travel patterns of serial burglars in committing their crimes. Other limited trials of the circle measurement, however, have found support for the principles of the circle measurement in the context of crimes of serial/sexual murder, rape, and arson *(19–21)*. Therefore, it would appear that the principles of the circle measurement are more applicable to crimes characterized by interpersonal violence, such as serial sexual murder, rape, and arson, rather than those featuring criminal enterprise and monetary gain such as that typically encountered in serial burglary.

Rate of Domocentricity

Having established in what circumstance the circle measurement can be applied, the next question is when can it be applied? As previously mentioned, the principles of the circle measurement operate on the premise of selecting the two furthest offense locations in hindsight, that is, after the commission of all offenses. However, in the context of an on-going investigation, how many offenses need to be committed before the offender demonstrates a domocentric movement pattern that may be predicted by the circle measure? Furthermore,

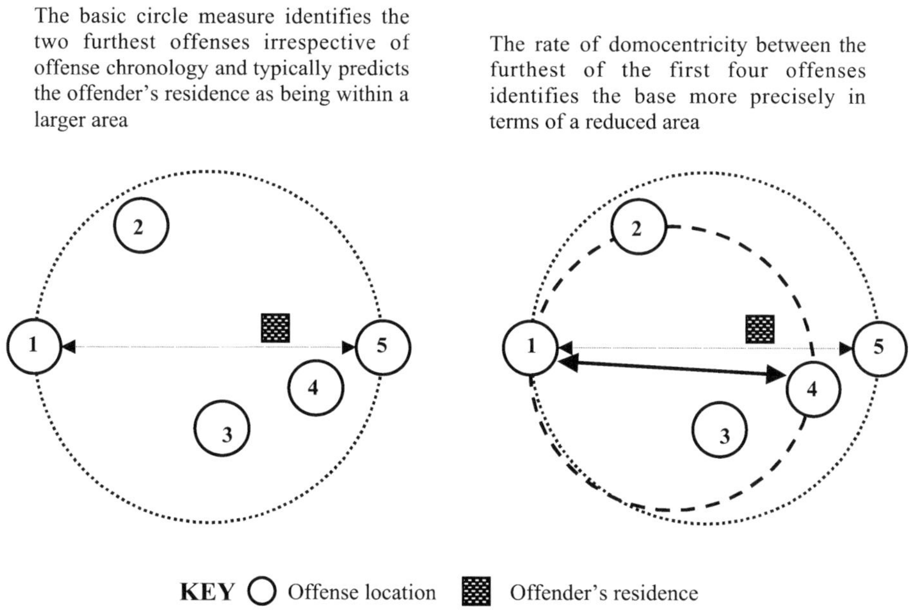

Fig. 10.3. Hypothetical examples of the basic circle measurement that predicts the location of the offender's residence based on the location of the two furthest offenses. However, the rate of domocentricity (ROD) allows for a more refined prediction after four offenses. Additionally, 69% of predictions based on the ROD have been found to be smaller than a prediction based on the basic circle measurement.

after determining what this offense rate may be, could predictions based on this minimum offense number also contribute to an accurate, yet reduced prediction area if later offenses *are not* taken into account?

In an effort to answer these questions, all offenses in each of the maps from the studies by Kocsis et al. *(17,18,20)* were compared with multiple diametric circles based on their commission in chronological order. The result of this experiment found that, on average, the circle measurement drawn from the two furthest offense locations of the first four offenses often encompassed the offender's residence. Additionally, it was found that the circle measurement taken from these locations produced an accurate, yet reduced area* in 69% of cases. Figure 10.3 provides a conceptual illustration of the application of the rate of domocentricity (ROD) principle.

*In comparison to the basic circle measure of the two furthest offenses in an entire offense series.

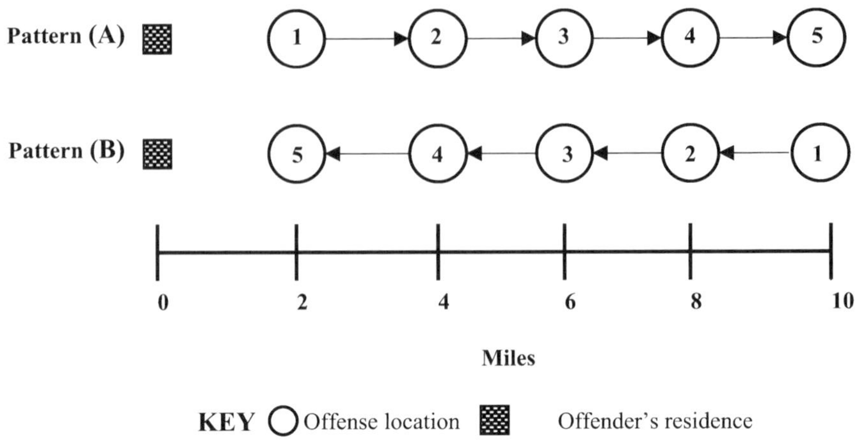

Fig. 10.4. Is there a pattern between the distances traveled to commit an offense and their sequence? If so, what is this pattern? Do offenders commit their initial offenses closer to their residence and progressively travel further away (pattern A) or do they commit their initial crimes further away and then progressively offend closer to home (pattern B)?

The practical use of the ROD is that the circle measurement can be applied, on average, after four offenses to predict an offender's likely area of residence. Furthermore, this prediction area is likely to be smaller than a prediction based on any combination of later offenses. As a final comment, however, it is crucial to remember that the ROD only applies to cases that demonstrate a domocentric movement pattern.

Distance Chronology

Another important consideration is whether there is any pattern in the distances offenders travel from their residences to commit a crime and the sequence in which these offenses occur. Do criminals commit their initial offense closer to their residence and then progressively travel further away, or are they more likely to commit their initial offense further away from their residence and then progressively commit crimes closer to their residence? Figure 10.4 provides a hypothetical illustration of these possible movement patterns.

Once again, these issues were considered in the context of the studies by Kocsis et al. *(17,18,20)* by measuring the distances between the location of each offense and the offender's residence, in the order in which each offense occurred. The results of this experiment suggested a general pattern whereby offenders tended to commit their initial crimes further away from their resi-

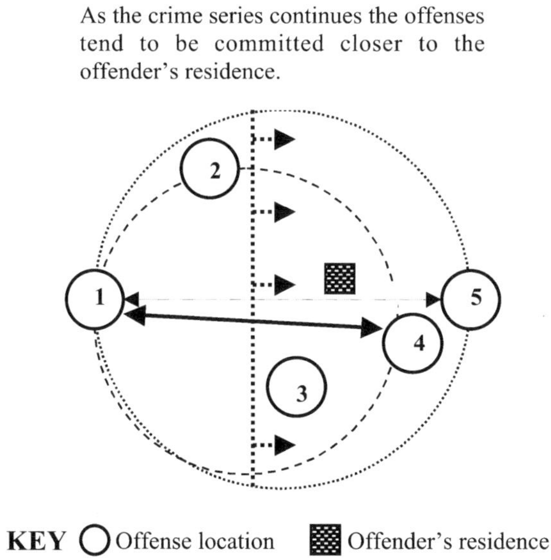

Fig. 10.5. The offense chronology trend indicates that initial offenses tend to be committed further away from the base and latter offenses closer to the offender's residence. This finding, in combination with the basic circle measurement and the rate of domocentricity, can assist in providing a further reduced area, as indicated by the small arrows pointing to the right.

dence and then progressively committed subsequent offenses closer to home (as illustrated in Fig. 10.4, pattern B). The value of this result is that in combination with the previously discussed principles, a further reduction in the prediction area can be approximated based on the sequence of the offense series. A hypothetical illustration of this appears in Fig. 10.5. The smaller circle prediction area identified by the ROD can be reduced to the area on the left of the circle because this is where later offenses are likely to occur and the research suggests may be closer to the offender's residence.

Developing a Geographic Profile

As discussed in the previous section, a number of important principles emerge from the studies conducted by Kocsis et al. *(17,18,20)* that endeavor to further refine the operation of the circle measurement, without the need to resort to any computerized geographic profiling system. The next part of this chapter is focused on creating an easy and accessible means for developing a geographic profile. This may be generated by the manual plotting of offense locations on a map accompanied by various simple measurements. It is these principles involved in developing such a geographic profile that will now be discussed via a series of simple, guiding steps.

Step 1: Suitability

It is important to exercise caution when evaluating the suitability of a crime for criminal profiling. One of the unfortunate problems in the contemporary practice of criminal profiling is the proclivity of some practitioners to overgeneralize and transpose research principles onto all manner of circumstance *(22)*. In the context of geographic profiling, it is crucial to remember that the principles that have been developed and canvassed in this chapter do not appear to be fully applicable to all forms of serial crime.* Although many principles appear to be useful in the context of crimes of interpersonal violence, such as serial/sexual murder, rape, and arson, which predominantly tend to follow a domocentric movement pattern in their commission, crimes related to aspects of criminal enterprise involving monetary gain do not appear to be so amenable. Consequently, the procedures outlined in this chapter for developing a geographic profile are not recommended for all crimes such as, for example, serial burglary.

It is equally important to remember that one of the primary assumptions underpinning geographic profiling is that the offender has a fixed place of residence. Consequently, these procedures are unlikely to be effective in the circumstance of an offender who adopts a transient lifestyle and who is thus unlikely to have a fixed place of abode.

Before embarking on the development of a geographic profile, it is important to establish that sufficient information is available. It should be apparent that the map-plotting and measurement principles underlying the development of a geographic profile require a number of locations for analysis. The issue of identifying suitable locations will be elaborated on shortly. Although the basic circle measurement is technically possible from simply two locations, as a general rule, it is not recommended that a geographic profile be developed when anything less than four locations are available for analysis.

Step 2: Verify and Identify Case Information

The strength of a geographic profile is dependent on the accuracy of the information being analyzed. If the case information is characterized by errors or omissions, then in all probability the value of a geographic profile derived

*It should be understood that applicability in this context relates to how reliable the principles are in accounting for an offender's movement patterns in the aforementioned studies.

from such material will be concomitantly compromised. Consequently, all case information with particular reference to offense locations, such as addresses and the chronology in which offenses occurred, should always be carefully verified.

Accepting that the case information is accurate it is equally important to ensure that all possible information is available. As demonstrated by the research in Chapter 4, the value of any criminal profile will be dependent on the case information available for analysis *(23)*. In the context of a geographic profile, case information will typically pertain to geographic locations relevant to the crime being examined. Consequently, it is important to satisfy oneself of two issues in particular for the development of a geographic profile.

First, have all locations relevant to the offense series been identified? In most circumstances this information will be readily discernible from, for example, the location of a structure that was burnt in an arson attack, or where the victim reports being assaulted in a rape. It is important, however, to be cognizant of ancillary locations that can also be used as potential coordinates in the development of a geographic profile. Although plotting the circle measurement requires as an absolute minimum, two spatial coordinates from which a diametric circle may be drawn, the ROD recommends a minimum of four coordinates. Consequently, an adequate number of coordinates should be available to generate even a rudimentary profile. Although in some circumstances additional coordinates may simply not be available, it is important to be mindful of other locations that may be of significance. For example, an assortment of coordinates can potentially be derived in the case of a murder from the location where the victim encountered the offender, where the victim was killed, where their body was deposited, or the location of an ATM machine where the offender withdrew funds using a credit card taken from the victim. Thus, in this hypothetical example of a murder four spatial locations/coordinates can be identified that have particular significance to the crime.

The second important type of information that should be ascertained for the purpose of developing a geographic profile is the chronological sequence of all incidents. This information should be collected at the larger macro-level of the individual offenses as well as at the smaller micro level of the sequence of differing events (such as those in the previous hypothetical example) that may occur within any particular offense.

Step 3: Mapping

Fundamental to the development of a geographic profile is the plotting of all locations on a map for easy reference. Consequently, a suitable map will need to be obtained that covers the region that the crimes under investigation have transpired within. This map should be sufficiently detailed to indicate street names as well as geographic and structural features, such as, but not limited to, rivers, bridges, train lines, and arterial routes for traffic.

With all relevant locations determined and a suitable map obtained, the logistical task of plotting each coordinate onto a map may then begin. Care should be taken to ensure that each coordinate is plotted clearly and as precisely as possible on the map. The chronology of each location should also be clearly recorded on the map. In the circumstance in which different types of locations are available (such as an initial attack location and a separate disposal site location for where a body is deposited) coding by the use of differing symbols or colors is very useful in indicating the differing types of information each location represents.

Step 4: Basic Circle Measurement

With all locations plotted on the map, the first measurement can be undertaken. As with all subsequent steps described herein, this measurement can be accomplished using basic geometry tools such as a ruler and a compass. Irrespective of the chronology of the plotted locations, identify the two furthest points on the map. Using the locations of these two points, draw a line connecting them. This line then forms the diameter of a circle that can be drawn with the aid of a compass, for example, on the map. The area within this circle on the map represents the initial prediction area of the geographic profile. This circle measurement provides a conceptual representation of the area within which the offender is likely to be operating with respect to the commission of their offenses. As discussed in the concluding section of this chapter, this prediction area can be used as a guide for determining where best to concentrate investigative efforts. In addition to providing a representation of the criminal activity area, the space within this initial circle measurement can also serve as a rudimentary prediction of the area within which the offender's residence may also be located.

Step 5: ROD

Following the initial circle measurement, the first four incident locations, as denoted by their chronology, should be identified. Having identified these four points, another diametric circle should be drawn using the two locations that are the furthest apart. This ROD measurement will have an approximately 66% probability of producing a smaller circle than that drawn by the basic circle measurement described in step 4, that may also encompass the offender's place of residence.

Step 6: Travel Clusters

To potentially focus the prediction area further, the overall distribution of all locations should be examined for any suggestion of clustering. Clustering will occur where offenses appear to be located in some general in close proximity to one another. If such a clustering pattern can be discerned, then the region within the circle measurement that is closest to this clustering may be of particular significance (*see* Fig. 10.5). In utilizing this procedure, one caveat must be expressed concerning its applicability. This procedure was developed from the findings of previous studies (e.g., refs. *17,18,20*) that suggested that a declining trend emerges in the distance an offender would be prepared to travel to commit subsequent offenses. It should, however, be understood that this trend is often gradual and thus may not be immediately apparent or readily manifest. Consequently, for this pattern to emerge, a reasonably high number of offenses are needed for this type of analysis.

Step 7: Environmental Considerations

In developing a geographic profile it is vital to also consider the physical environment when appraising the prediction areas identified by the measurements. In particular, it is important to be cognizant of the inappropriateness of including any type of uninhabitable terrain in the prediction area of a geographic profile. Areas within a map denoted by terrain types such as, but not limited to, lakes, rivers, oceans, or desert to name a few can generally be discounted and thus excluded from the prediction area of a geographic profile.

Step 8: Adjustments

In developing a criminal profile, it is generally important to remain flexible and keep an open mind by, for example, re-evaluating any new information relative to the case. The development of a geographic profile should not be based on the static evaluation of information. Consequently, should any further information become available, such as, for example, evidence concerning another offense, then the various plotting procedures and measurements in developing a geographic profile will need to be undertaken afresh, to incorporate the new information.

Step 9: Interpretation

The information or prediction of a geographic profile is represented by the areas on the map encapsulated by the various plotted measurements previously discussed. However, two important principles underpin the interpretation of these measurements. First, interpretation should always be approached on the basis of prioritization and not elimination. Second, the areas encapsulated by the various measurements on a map represent the prediction areas (plural) of a geographic profile.

As a mechanism to potentially improve the perspicuity of a geographic profile the various measures described in this chapter cumulatively attempt to reduce the total size of the measured area in any map and thus help focus the profile. This focusing process is principally accomplished by identifying regions where the various measurements overlap one another. When the various measurement principles are combined together there will often emerge a region, typically the smallest in size to all separate measurements, that can be discerned by its overlap with all measured areas (*see* Fig. 10.5 as a hypothetical example). This reduced region identified by the combined overlaps of all measurements does **not** represent the geographic profile but merely one single component of it.

By following this interpretative principle of prioritization, any reduced region identified by such overlaps represents the area in respect of which attention should be initially focused because of it possibly encompassing the offender's residence. It is important to note that the regions outside of this overlapping area, which are still encapsulated by any number of separate measurements or fewer overlaps, are also part of the geographic profile and represent other prediction areas possibly containing the offender's residence. However, these areas should occupy a descending order of priority based on the number of overlapping measurements. Additionally, it is crucial for readers to appreciate that these various areas of overlap will not necessarily appear in a symmetrically centralized region relative to the areas depicted by the various measurements. Although these areas of overlap may, in some circumstances, possess a discernibly centripetal position (such as that depicted, for example, in Fig. 10.5) they can also emerge in an eccentric location relative to the measurements and should not therefore be arbitrarily dismissed as irrelevant.

In identifying and isolating the prediction areas it is important to bear in mind that the various measurements use simple geometric shapes as theoretical approximations of profiling principles. The purpose of these simplified shapes is to facilitate the user-friendly application of these profiling principles. Accordingly, the various borders depicted by the plotting of these measurements should not be treated as magical lines beyond which other investigative considerations are not warranted. Any area that shares some reasonably discernible proximity with a border should remain within the scope of consideration. A hypothetical example will be used to better illustrate this point. A suspect who resides in a neighboring street just outside of a prediction area should not be eliminated from consideration. Instead the proximity of their location to this measurement should be regarded as a potential link to the prediction areas of the geographic profile.

Investigative Applications of a Geographic Profile

Having discussed the theoretical origins, the development of research principles, and the procedures involved in developing a geographic profile, it seems appropriate to conclude the chapter with some discussion on how the information forming a geographic profile can be used to assist in a criminal investigation. It is imperative to always bear in mind that a geographic profile should always be used as a method of prioritizing an investigation. That is, the prediction areas of a geographic profile should only be used as a mechanism to prioritize options concerning how a criminal investigation should proceed; it should not be used to eliminate options altogether. In this way, investigative leads that demonstrate some connection to the area denoted by a geographic profile can be given prioritization over those, for example, that do not demonstrate such a nexus. A prediction area should therefore only be used as a mechanism for prioritizing and focusing investigative efforts. It should not under any circumstance be used as a mechanism to disregard potential leads.

Although there are numerous circumstantial contexts in which information contained in a geographic profile may be applied to a criminal investigation *(24)*, these circumstances can typically be broken down into two generic types of application: proactive or reactive. An explanation of each appears below.

Pro-Active Applications

The term *pro-active* in the context of applying a geographic profile refers to its application in initiating some type of investigative and/or policing strategy that may potentially deter further offenses and/or actively generate further investigative leads. In pro-active applications of a geographic profile, the information derived from the profile is typically focused on providing an indication of an offender's area of criminal activity as denoted, for example, by the basic circle measurement (*see* step 4). An example of a pro-active application of a geographic profile is its use in identifying a region for the purpose of canvassing the community in an area to gain further information and thereby additional investigative leads. Another example, involves the deployment of policing units to particular areas to potentially deter and/or apprehend an offender in the commission of a crime. With a general area defined as being one where an offender may commit offenses, police patrols can be deployed to that area and thus act as a potential inhibitor to the commission of further offenses. Similarly, stakeout operations can be initiated in those areas where an offender is thought to reside or frequent. A classic illustration of this tactic involved the investigation into the Atlanta child murders. In that case, investigators had determined that the offender was dumping the corpses of murder victims into main waterways. Thus, stakeouts of the bridges spanning the waterways were initiated. From one of these stakeouts a license plate number was identified when a car was seen suspiciously crossing the bridge that eventually led to the apprehension of the offender *(25)*.

Reactive Applications

In contrast to pro-active applications, reactive applications of a geographic profile tend to be more oriented toward prioritizing leads and investigative options. One example of the application of a geographic profile in a reactive context is in cross-referencing matches between the prediction areas of a geographic profile and the addresses of suspects. Suspects whose addresses are located within prediction areas can be prioritized over those whose address is located outside a prediction area. Geographic profiles can also be used in a similar fashion for the generation of new suspects by similar cross-referencing between the prediction area of a geographic profile and various relevant databases. An example of this application is where a specific model of car was observed leaving a crime scene. By accessing a motor registry database, a cross-referencing exercise can be undertaken whereby all registered owners of the particular model of car who are also located in the geographic profile prediction area can be identified and prioritized for investigative purposes *(24)*. Another reactive application of a geographic profile is in the collection of forensic evidence. Although the advent of DNA trace evidence has revolutionized the way individuals can be associated with a crime, the collection and analysis of matching DNA samples currently remains a costly endeavor. In this respect, geographic profiles can be used to focus the number of samples collected and thus potentially reduce investigation costs. For example, in some instances, investigations have involved large-scale DNA samples drawn from a community in the hope of obtaining a sample that matches DNA evidence obtained from a crime scene. With the use of a geographic profile the collection of such samples from the community can be first prioritized to include only those located within the prediction areas of the profile *(24)*.

CONCLUSION

Some indication of the area in which an unknown criminal's residence is likely to be found is a potentially valuable piece of information to any investigation. This information, however, should never be relied on to the exclusion of other information. Rather, it should be used in conjunction with other information typically contained in a criminal profile that also describes the probable offender's characteristics. Geographic considerations only represent one facet of information useful to investigators. The usefulness of the information contained in any criminal profile is more likely to be maximized when all facets of information are logically integrated together. Only through the development of a holistic picture of the probable offender will investigators be able to realize the potential of a criminal profile. Thus, geographic profiles should always be regarded as simply one subcomponent of a criminal profile.

This chapter has discussed the origins of geographic profiling as well as the focus and limitations of available research in the area. These limitations largely prompted CAP research that has sought to develop a means for developing a geographic profile through manual plotting and measurement of various locations on a map. In this respect, CAP research primarily attempts to build on the basic principles of the circle measurement in a manner that allows for its application in a practical context, such as in the circumstance of an ongoing criminal investigation. This chapter endeavors to articulate the findings of CAP research into a series of simple, easy-to-follow procedural steps. It is hoped that these steps will serve as a useful guide for investigators to follow when considering the offense locations of an offender without needing to resort to commercially marketed computer programs for geographic profiling. It should be understood, however, that akin to most manual endeavors, practice will be required in the proficient application of these principles.

REFERENCES

1. Brantingham, P.L. and Brantingham, P.J. (1981). Environmental criminology. Beverly Hills, CA: Sage.
2. Reppetto, T.A. (1974). Residential crime. Cambridge, MA: Ballinger.
3. Rengert, G.F. and Wasilchick, J. (1985). Suburban burglary. Springfield, IL: Charles C. Thomas.
4. Fisher, A.J. (1993). Techniques of crime scene investigation, 5th ed. New York: Elsevier.
5. Frank, G. (1966). The Boston strangler. New York: New American Library.
6. Kind, S.S. (1987). Navigational ideas and the Yorkshire Ripper investigation. Journal of Navigation, 40, 385–393.

7. Levine, N. (2000). Crimestat: A spatial statistics program for the analysis of crime incident locations (version 1.1). National Institute of Justice: Washington, DC.
8. Rossmo, D.K. (1996). Targeting victims: Serial killers and the urban environment. In: O'Reilly-Fleming, T., ed. Serial and mass murder. Toronto: Canadian Scholars Press, pp.133–154.
9. Young, G. (2003, August). Mapping mayhem: The geography of crime. Computerage.
10. Palermo, G.B. and Kocsis, R.N. (2005). Offender profiling: An introduction to the sociopsychological analysis of violent crime. Springfield IL: CC Thomas.
11. Snook, B., Canter, D.V., Bennell, C. (2002). Predicting the home location of serial offenders: A preliminary comparison of the accuracy of human judges with a geographic profiling system. Behavioral Science and Law, 20, 109–118.
12. Canter, D.V. and Larkin, P. (1993). The environmental range of serial rapists. Journal of Environmental Psychology, 13, 63–69.
13. Groth, N.A., Burgess, A.W., Holmstrom, L.L. (1977). Rape: Power, anger and sexuality. American Journal of Psychiatry, 134, 1239–1243.
14. Hickey, E.W. (1997). Serial murderers and their victims, 2nd ed. Fresno, CA: Wadsworth.
15. Ressler, R.K., Burgess, A., Douglas, J.E. (1988). Sexual homicide: Patterns and motives. New York: Lexington Books.
16. Canter, D.V., Coffey, T., Huntley, M., Missen, C. (2000). Predicting serial killers home base using a decision support system. Journal of Quantitative Criminology, 16(4), 16–31.
17. Kocsis, R.N. and Irwin, H.J. (1997). An analysis of spatial patterns in serial rape, arson and burglary: The utility of the circle theory of environmental range for psychological profiling. Psychiatry, Psychology and Law, 4, 195–206.
18. Kocsis, R.N., Cooksey, R.W., Irwin, H.J., Allen, G. (2002). A further assessment of "Circle Theory" for geographic psychological profiling. Australian and New Zealand Journal of Criminology, 35(1), 43–62.
19. Godwin, G.M. and Canter, D.V. (1997). Encounter and death: The spatial behavior of U.S. serial killers. Policing: An International Journal of Strategy and Management, 20(1), 24–38.
20. Kocsis, R. N. (1995). An empirical assessment of the spatial offense patterns of the Sydney Granny Killer. Unpublished research project.
21. Lundrigan, S. and Canter, D.V. (2001). A multivariate analysis of serial murderers disposal site location choice. Journal of Environmental Psychology, 21, 423–432.
22. Kocsis, R.N. and Palermo, G.B. (2005). Ten major problems with criminal profiling. American Journal of Forensic Psychiatry, 26(2), 1–26.
23. Kocsis, R.N., Heller, G.Z., Try, A. (2003). Visual vs. narrative case material: Their impact on criminal psychological profiling? International Journal of Offender Therapy and Comparative Criminology, 47(6), 664–676.
24. Rossmo, D.K. (1995). Place, space, and police investigation: Hunting serial violent criminals. In: Eck, J.E. and Weisburd, D.A., eds. Crime and place: Crime prevention studies. Monsey, NY: Criminal Justice Press, pp. 217–235.
25. Douglas, J.E. and Oleshaker, M. (1995). Mindhunter. New York: Scribner.

Chapter 11

Procedural Considerations and Format Guidelines

Summary

Although a person engaged in developing a criminal profile may conceive many valuable ideas and insights concerning the probable offender of a crime, this information can be wasted or even compromised if not communicated properly. Consequently, the purpose of this chapter is to outline a series of professional, ethical, and procedural considerations that are recommended for the development of a criminal profile in the form of a written report.

Key Words: Criminal profile; written reports; ethical and procedural considerations.

Introduction

In essence, a criminal profile represents a form of expert opinion that is provided by one party to another party who seeks an opinion concerning the likely perpetrator(s) of a crime or series of crimes. This chapter focuses on how to write a criminal profile. The information that comprises a criminal profile is typically communicated in either a verbal or written form. In the verbal form, items of information constituting a profile are simply communicated to investigators in circumstances such as a face-to-face meeting. An advantage of this method is the expediency in communication between the investigator(s) and the individual consulted for the purpose of developing a criminal profile. Additionally, verbal communication readily facilitates an exchange of information should elaboration on any specific point be required. A disadvantage of criminal profiles being furnished in this way, however, is that there is far greater potential for misinterpretation and/or misunderstanding. Additionally, criminal profiles provided in verbal form tend to lack

From: *Criminal Profiling: Principles and Practice*
By: R. N. Kocsis © Humana Press Inc., Totowa, NJ

accountability in terms of subsequent verification, should this become necessary, which can in turn raise questions surrounding the professional credibility of the individual providing the information or indeed the profile itself.

The second, and arguably more common method of communicating a criminal profile, is in the form of a report. The length, form, and content of such reports vary considerably and are dependent on the nature of the matter under consideration as well as the individual consulted to develop the criminal profile. In many respects, criminal profiles communicated in the written form are the inverse of those communicated in verbal form. An advantage of written profiles is the increased potential for content verification at a later point in time and thus greater accountability. Arguably, the written form minimizes the potential for misunderstanding the information contained in a profile. Furthermore, written profiles can easily and more faithfully be distributed to any number of persons with a reduced risk of distortion occurring via dissemination. Unfortunately, a disadvantage of written profiles is that they often take longer to produce and are therefore, comparatively speaking, lacking in expediency when compared with verbal profiles. Additionally, there is a somewhat reduced capacity for immediate clarification of an issue should it be required. Although a variety of logistical circumstances may arise that necessitate the communication of a profile by verbal means, a criminal profile in the form of a formal report is preferable. Unfortunately, however, the time-conscious nature of our world will not always allow for the development of a written profile. Consequently, it is always best in the event that a verbal profile is required to follow this up at the earliest possible juncture with a written report, if only for your own file in the event that a written report is not required by a commissioning person or agency.

Before describing the recommended structure and format of a criminal profile, there are a number of procedural and ethical issues that should be considered before one embarks on the development of a criminal profile. The following observations are not provided in any particular order indicative of their importance.

Availability

First, ensure that adequate time is available to undertake the composition of a profile in a competent and professional manner. A consultation should first consider when a profile is due and assess the time needed to evaluate the case information available and whether there is sufficient time in which to competently undertake this task in view of any competing commitments. If there is insufficient time in which to evaluate the case material and construct a profile, the task should not be embarked on and should instead be deferred to another consultant. To embark on a professional task knowing that there is insufficient time to provide a competent product is arguably unprofessional and detrimental to one's reputation as well as that of profiling in general.

Due Diligence

Closely aligned to availability should be a work ethic of diligence in attending to the matter in a timely fashion. When engaging in the type of critical evaluation inherent to the analysis and development of a criminal profile it is imperative that the work be undertaken in a totally focused manner. The matter in question should be the only issue under consideration in the time specifically allocated for the task.

Environment

Congruent with the previous principle of diligence is the environment in which such work should be undertaken. The environment should, wherever possible, be devoid of distractions, competing commitments, and other potential interruptions that may hamper or impede the evaluation of the matter. A private office or study where noise can be minimized is preferable for producing the best possible results and also for reasons of privacy and security.

Confidentiality

Confidentiality in handling case materials provided to you for examination should be of paramount importance at all times. In most instances the issue of confidentiality will be stipulated by the consulting agency. Nonetheless, it cannot be emphasized enough that the handling of case material relating to an on-going investigation must be treated with the strictest of confidentiality. Often personal, identifying information will be part and parcel of such material and this should not be disseminated to any third parties without prior approval from the consulting organization. (Indeed, it is recommended that such authorization always be obtained in writing before any disclosure.) Naturally, issues of confidentiality apply not only to the handling of case material, but also to any communications with third parties relating to the matter or consultancy, such as, for example, journalists seeking to report the crime.

These issues of confidentiality should be followed not only during the course of an investigation but thereafter also. The only conceivable exception to these confidentiality provisions is when the pertinent information has legally appeared in the public domain, such as at the conclusion of a trial following a public hearing and sentencing. Even within this circumstance, however, it is advisable as a professional courtesy to inform the consulting organization of any planned dissemination or use of materials originally obtained during the course of a consultancy.

Professional Courtesy

It is important to acknowledge the boundaries of one's own professional expertise and concurrently recognize the expertise of other professionals within the field of criminal profiling or in other disciplines who may possess greater expertise and experience in a given area. When confronted by a request for a criminal profile pertaining to an issue that is not within the typical scope of one's expertise it is important to possess the professionalism to suggest the matter be referred to another who may genuinely be able to achieve a better outcome owing to their particular expertise and experience.

Objectivity

When developing a criminal profile, it is important to remain independent and objective at all times. Circumstances typically requiring a criminal profile involve an investigative organization consulting an external party to obtain some new or different insight into an unsolved crime. In light of this circumstance therefore it is important to adopt a position of independent objectivity; to do otherwise often defeats the purpose of the consultancy in seeking to potentially obtain new insight and perspective into a crime or crime series.

Accordingly, when developing a profile it is crucial to maintain a degree of professional distance from the consulting organization. Specifically, the evaluation of the matter and the development of a criminal profile must be carried out in an objective manner with all conclusions supported and reported in a methodical fashion. It is recommended that any consideration of an existing hypothesis concerning the matter originally nominated by the consulting organization or another party should only occur after one's own independent evaluation of the case material has been completed, so as not to color or influence one's own assessment of the matter.

In a similar manner, the conclusions articulated in a criminal profile should always be made in a completely objective capacity akin to those opined by more traditional experts. Hypothetically, therefore, all conclusions arrived at within a criminal profile should not alter according to the commissioning agency. That is, conclusions reached should be the same irrespective of whether the request to compile the profile was made by an investigating/prosecuting organization or some opposing party (such as, for example, a defense counsel in the same matter). Indeed, should the conclusions of a profile come to be tested in court, answers to questions posed in this forum should be objectively provided irrespective of whether such answers assist or detract from the arguments mounted by the party who originally commissioned the profile.

A final issue related to objectivity concerns the quality of case material available for examination. A consultation should ideally be undertaken only after all case material held by the consulting organization has been supplied, not just a selection of material that the organization elects to provide. Although limited argument exists to support the select release of case material, the adoption of such a practice, unfortunately, is prone to compromise the value of the criminal profile generated from a consideration of this portion of the material and indeed can result in bias owing to the artificial quarantining of potentially important information. Consequently, whenever possible, the development of a criminal profile should be undertaken with the benefit of all relevant case material currently available to the commissioning person/organization.

Integrity

A position of integrity should always be adopted when discharging a legal duty and in this sense undertaking a consultancy for the purpose of compiling a criminal profile is no exception. Any work undertaken in this context should represent the consultant's own honest and uninfluenced opinion concerning the matter. Consequently, the development of a criminal profile should only be undertaken in circumstances in which no undue or inappropriate influence on the consultant exists and no conflicts of interests arise. In a similar fashion, therefore, the communication of a criminal profile should always, whenever possible, be made in a transparent and verifiable manner. In most cases this will involve the construction of a written report (the recommended method will be discussed shortly), which may in turn be subsequently open to independent scrutiny.

Professionalism

The development of a criminal profile should only ever be undertaken for a professional purpose. The relationship between the consultant and that of the organization or person requesting the criminal profile should be one of professional purpose and not originate through any informal personal relationship that may exist between the parties because this can lead to conflicts of interest or at least, perceived conflicts. Although collegiality is a healthy dynamic in many work environments, the provision of a criminal profile on any informal basis that is not related to a professional request is not recommended. Any consultation undertaken outside a professionally grounded interaction is bound to be regarded with suspicion concerning the objectivity and integrity of a criminal profile developed in such circumstances. For this reason, when developing a criminal profile, care should always be taken to acknowledge the commissioning party from the outset. This should also be accompanied by a description of the agreed scope of the criminal profile, time frames, and any questions specifically posed. In most circumstances it is not recommended that a consultation be undertaken in a purely *gratis* capacity because such circumstances are prone to potential questions concerning factors of personal favor, which once again detract from the objectivity and therefore credibility of the profile provided.

Format Guidelines for Written Profiles

The circumstances that may warrant the use of a criminal profile in a criminal investigation vary considerably. Consequently, the format of a written criminal profile may vary in that it will largely be dependent on the nature and circumstances of the particular case under examination as well as the specific issues prompting the consultation in the first place. Nonetheless, to assist in developing a criminal profile the following principles should be observed when compiling a written profile.

Possibly the most fundamental general principle is that any report constituting a criminal profile must be clearly legible and articulate, observing correct grammar, spelling, and syntax. A report constituting a criminal profile should always be typed. Thus, hand-written profiles should be avoided. Second, reports should also avoid the unnecessary use of jargon, clichés, colloquialisms, or slang unless appropriate to the circumstances, such as for example, when quoting graffiti or words communicated during the course of a crime or in repeating the exact words of a witness, an interviewed suspect, and so on. A report should, wherever possible, be written in a formal and impartial tone that aims to objectively assess all available case material. Third, all pages in a report should be clearly numbered. Concomitantly, some small text header or footer should appear on all pages of the report so as to identify the document, the matter it was written in reference to, and the author. It is also a good idea to include a paragraph numbering sequence in one margin throughout the entire report thereby allowing any reader to readily identify and if necessary, reference any specific portion of the report. So as not to detract from the overall structure and headings used in a report, the use of

DR RICHARD N. KOCSIS
B.A. (Hons)., *Psych.* Cert. Man., M.CRIM., Ph.D. *Psych.*
FORENSIC PSYCHOLOGIST

Street Number & Name, Suburb
City, State, Zip Code, Country
Ph/Fax XXXX XXXXX Email XXXX

XX May XXXX

Captain John Smith
Homicide Squad
Criminal Investigation Division
MM Police Department
City, State, Zip Code
Country

Dear Captain Smith,

Re: Homicide Offense Series (Dates – Dates)

[1] Thank you for electing to consult me for the purpose of developing a criminal profile that may be of assistance to your homicide investigation.

Box 11.1. Hypothetical report referral details.

italics, bold, underline, highlighting, and other means of distinguishing text should be kept to a minimum. Finally, written reports should not under any circumstance be written as a single continuous block of writing. Instead, the report should be systematically broken down into discrete sections that a reader can easily identify and refer to.

Having canvassed these general principles a number of thematic sections are suggested.

Step 1: Report Referral Details

Akin to any form of expert report, a criminal profile should begin by clearly identifying what the report is in reference to. Thus, a profile* should commence on a page bearing an identifying letterhead as well as any relevant contact details. The report should start by addressing the person(s) from the consulting organization who requested the criminal profile. These particulars should then be followed by some form of reference details that clearly identifies the matter to which the report refers as well as some description of the nature of the report commissioned. As a professional courtesy it is suggested that the report commence with a brief statement thanking the organization for their decision in selecting you to prepare a criminal profile. An example appears in Box 11.1.

*Please note that the term *profile* and *report* are used interchangeably in this chapter.

Step 2: Opening Caveat

Early in the report, ideally immediately after the referral details, a statement should be made clearly advising the reader of the potential limitations of the opinions expressed in the report and criminal profiles in general. It should be emphasized that criminal profiles should only be relied on as a supplement to a criminal investigation and in this sense may be used to augment existing investigative lines of inquiry. Therefore, potential or established leads or suspects should never be dismissed on the basis of apparent or perceived incongruity with the conclusions articulated in the profile. Ideally, a criminal profile should only be used as a conduit to assist in prioritizing options. In this respect, a criminal profile should be thought of as a means of aiding an investigation and not as a purely reductive mechanism. An example of such a caveat appears in Box 11.2.

Step 3: Itemized Information List

Following the referral details and opening caveat, it is advisable to include an itemized list detailing all material supplied and considered in compiling the criminal profile. The creation of such a list supports the professional credibility of the report by clearly accounting for all information that was relied on in the formulation of the profile. In most instances, this will involve systematically listing the materials contained in the brief of evidence supplied by the consulting organization. In addition to such material, notations should also be made of any other form of information that may have been relied on in drawing conclusions articulated in the profile. Consequently, information, such as, but not limited to, additional conversations concerning the matter or interviews with relevant parties involved with the investigation of the matter should be noted. A limited example of such a list appears in Box 11.3.

Step 4: Case Summary

The case summary represents the first substantial component of the report. The purpose of a case summary is to provide the reader with a systematic and thorough description of the apparent events or facts concerning the matter as derived from the materials supplied and enumerated in the previous case information list.

In most instances, the materials compiled by a police investigation consist of a large assortment of documents including, but not limited to, witness statements, forensic reports, and photographic materials. Most investigative personnel are trained to gather and assemble relevant case information to form a legal brief of evidence. The purpose of a case summary is to piece together

DR RICHARD N. KOCSIS
B.A. (Hons)., *Psych.* Cert. Man., M.CRIM., Ph.D. *Psych.*
FORENSIC PSYCHOLOGIST

Street Number & Name, Suburb
City, State, Zip Code, Country
Ph/Fax XXXX XXXXX Email XXXX

XX May XXXX

Captain John Smith
Homicide Squad
Criminal Investigation Division
MM Police Department
City, State, Zip Code
Country

Dear Captain Smith,

Re: Homicide Offense Series (Dates – Dates)

[1] Thank you for electing to consult me for the purpose of developing a criminal profile that may be of assistance to your homicide investigation.

[2] From the outset I feel it important to stress that the information contained in this report should not be exclusively relied upon for the co-ordination of your investigation. Rather, it should be considered as an aid in considering and exploring possibilities in your investigation as well as prioritizing the relevance of existing leads. Under no circumstance should the information provided in this report be used to dismiss information or disregard potential leads gathered during the course of your investigation.

Box 11.2. Caveat statement. The caveat statement appears in larger font.

DR RICHARD N. KOCSIS
B.A. (Hons)., *Psych.* Cert. Man., M.CRIM., Ph.D. *Psych.*
FORENSIC PSYCHOLOGIST

Street Number & Name, Suburb
City, State, Zip Code, Country
Ph/Fax XXXX XXXXX Email XXXX

XX May XXXX

Captain John Smith
Homicide Squad
Criminal Investigation Division
MM Police Department
City, State, Zip Code
Country

Dear Captain Smith,

Re: Homicide Offense Series (Dates – Dates)

[1] Thank you for electing to consult me for the purpose of developing a criminal profile that may be of assistance to your homicide investigation.

[2] From the outset I feel it important to stress that the information contained in this report should not be exclusively relied upon for the co-ordination of your investigation. Rather, it should be considered as an aid in considering and exploring possibilities in your investigation as well as prioritizing the relevance of existing leads. Under no circumstance should the information provided in this report be used to dismiss information or disregard potential leads gathered during the course of your investigation.

[3] My assessment of these matters is based on my evaluation of the following materials:

- Statement of Patrol officer P. Brown MM Police Department, dated XX/XX/XXXX
- Statement of Det. G. White, MM Police Department, dated XX/XX/XXXX
- Second statement of Det. G.White MM Police Department, dated XX/XX/XXXX
- Statement of Officer A. Blue, Crime Scene Investigation Unit, MM Police Department, dated XX/XX/XXXX
- Statement of Officer B. Black, Crime Scene Investigation Unit, MM Police Department, dated XX/XX/XXXX
- Forensic evidence reports of Officers A. Blue & B. Black, Crime, Crime Scene Investigation Unit, MM Police Department, dated XX/XX/XXXX
- Report of Ms. S. Yellow, County Coroner dated XX/XX/XXXX
- Autopsy report of Dr. P. Wells, Medical Examiner, MM County Morgue.
- Forensic Entomologist report of Dr. K. Blanley, University of XXXXXXXXXX

Box 11.3. Itemized list of information/materials. The materials list appears in larger font.

all of the individual items of information contained in the case materials and provide an easily comprehensible narrative summarizing all relevant and available information concerning the matter. Thus, the case summary should synthesize all the information contained in the original case materials in a coherent fashion.

The inclusion of a case summary is advantageous for a number of reasons and is accordingly recommended. A case summary is an excellent way for the consultant profiler to familiarize themselves with the material by thoroughly reading all the available information surrounding the matter. In this respect, the case summary also serves as a demonstration of the consulting profiler's understanding of the case information. The case summary also serves as an excellent reference source for a reader wishing to consider the relevance of any reasoning, conclusions, or comments required in subsequent sections of the report.

The size and structure of a case summary is dependent on the nature of the matter(s) under consideration. Accordingly, only a number of generic principles can be suggested in constructing a case summary. Naturally, should the matter under consideration relate to only a small number of incidents, the extent of the case summary may be significantly less than a matter involving a greater number of offenses or incidents.

A case summary should only be based on the source material forming the itemized list of information. Consequently, information should not be included in a case summary that does not have some identifiable source or reference to at least one of the items listed in the information list. It must be remembered that the case summary represents an objective and readily comprehensible summation of the information as discerned from the case materials. Therefore, it is important to avoid infusing this summation of the available case information with interpretations or conclusions concerning what various items of information may or may not suggest. The synthesis of such ideas should only occur later in the report. A limited hypothetical example of a case summary appears in Box 11.4.

Step 5: Evaluation

As stated previously, the case summary of a report should objectively summarize the available case information without comment as to what the information may suggest. Instead, it is recommended that a separate section be specifically devoted to the interpretation of this information and the provision of a descriptive profile of the probable offender(s). Consequently, a report should present a case summary section followed by an evaluation section. The respective themes of the two sections should be readily distinguishable

DR RICHARD N. KOCSIS
B.A. (Hons)., *Psych.* Cert. Man., M.CRIM., Ph.D. *Psych.*
FORENSIC PSYCHOLOGIST

Street Number & Name, Suburb
City, State, Zip Code, Country
Ph/Fax XXXX XXXXX Email XXXX

XX May XXXX

Captain John Smith
Homicide Squad
Criminal Investigation Division
MM Police Department
City, State, Zip Code
Country

Dear Captain Smith,

Re: Homicide Offense Series (Dates – Dates)

[1] Thank you for electing to consult me for the purpose of developing a criminal profile that may be of assistance to your homicide investigation.

[2] From the outset I feel it important to stress that the information contained in this report should not be exclusively relied upon for the co-ordination of your investigation. Rather, it should be considered as an aid in considering and exploring possibilities in your investigation as well as prioritizing the relevance of existing leads. Under no circumstance should the information provided in this report be used to dismiss information or disregard potential leads gathered during the course of your investigation.

[3] My assessment of these matters is based on my evaluation of the following materials:

- Statement of Patrol officer P. Brown MM Police Department, dated XX/XX/XXXX
- Statement of Det. G. White, MM Police Department, dated XX/XX/XXXX
- Second statement of Det. G.White MM Police Department, dated XX/XX/XXXX
- Statement of Officer A. Blue, Crime Scene Investigation Unit, MM Police Department, dated XX/XX/XXXX
- Statement of Officer B. Black, Crime Scene Investigation Unit, MM Police Department, dated XX/XX/XXXX
- Forensic evidence reports of Officers A. Blue & B. Black, Crime, Crime Scene Investigation Unit, MM Police Department, dated XX/XX/XXXX
- Report of Ms. S. Yellow, County Coroner dated XX/XX/XXXX
- Autopsy report of Dr. P. Wells, Medical Examiner, MM County Morgue.
- Forensic Entomologist report of Dr. K. Blanley, University of XXXXXXXXXX
-

==//==

[4] My assessment of these crimes will begin with an objective summation of the evidence, as discerned from the material currently available to me and as detailed above. This summation will be followed by an evaluation of each of these crimes and the possible offender followed in turn by suggestions on how your investigation may proceed in order to apprehend the offender(s). I will in addition address each of your questions in turn.

Case Summary

[5] *Offense (1) – Murder of Ms. T. Gray found on XX/XX/XXXX*

On Tuesday the XX of May XXXX at approximately XXpm Officer F. Green based at the MM Police station received a call from a citizen by the name of Mr. P Broody who reported finding a nude body whilst walking his dog in the XX Park. Patrol officer P. Brown was dispatched to Mr. Broody's location where he confirmed the presence of a corpse, immediately cordoned off the area and called for back-up and investigative personnel. In response to this call an investigative team was assembled to examine the crime scene. The body was determined to be that of a Caucasian female later identified as Ms T Gray, a 20 year old sophomore student at the neighbouring XXXXX college. Her body was completely nude with the exception of a gold colored bracelet found on her left ankle. The body was found in a supine position in the outlying area of an open walking park. Whilst the body was completely unclothed it was nonetheless extensively covered by branches and other foliage. Forensic examination of the crime scene and Ms. Gray's body could not locate any relevant hair or fibre evidence. A post-mortem examination of Ms. Gray's body revealed her mode of death as being by ligature strangulation owing to bruising and minor lacerations around her neck. Forensic entomological examination of the corpse indicate that Ms. Gray's body may have been secreted in this location for up to XXX days prior to its discovery. ……….

Box 11.4. Case summary. The case summary appears in larger font.

to the reader. That is, the case summary should be an objective summation of the case information, whereas the case evaluation should interpret the case material in a way that offers the consultant profiler's view of the case.

Again, the material inherent to this section will be very much dependent on the nature and circumstances of the matter under consideration as well as any issues specifically posed to the profiler. The evaluation will represent a combination of logical and critical analysis of the case information with reference to any pertinent research. Again, a number of generic rules should be observed. First, the evaluation should be written in a format that is easy to follow and succinct. Thus, the section should articulate systematically thoughts and conclusions. An evaluation should not, for example, merely present a series of disjointed sentences articulating various hypotheses. Rather, the information should be linked in a clear, concise, and easy-to-follow narrative.

Second, the evaluation should always be as comprehensive as possible. The evaluation should incorporate all information concerning the biographical and geographical aspects concerning the probable offender(s). In the presentation of this material, it is recommended that the biographical material be canvassed first, followed, where appropriate, by any geographical information. As indicated in the previous chapter, the processes for developing a geographic profile will often necessitate the plotting of a map. Consequently, it is suggested that the report discuss the conclusions reached from plotting the map within the evaluation section. For example, the profile should describe regions or suburbs that were identified by the map as encompassing the offender's likely residence. In providing this information clear references should also be made to the map so that such conclusions can be referenced and verified by the reader. Naturally, this procedure will also entail the inclusion of a copy of the map with the report. Any such map, however, should only be attached as an appendix to the report. Once again, a limited hypothetical example of such a case evaluation is provided in Box 11.5.

Step 6: Investigative Application(s)

The evaluation section is designed to articulate the consultant profiler's interpretation of the matter. Thus, features such as the characteristics of the probable offender(s) should be fully described in this section of the report. However, it is recommended that another separate section, entitled, for example, "Investigative Applications," be devoted to discussing how this information may be applied in some practical context by investigators.

The scope of this material will be very much dependent on the circumstances of the matter under consideration in addition to the ingenuity of the consultant profiler in conceiving of legally viable options for further explora-

Evaluation

[9] From my consideration of the information made available to me in this matter the murders of Ms. Gray, Ms. Red and Ms. Orange were in my view, most likely all committed by a single Caucasian male somewhere in the age range of mid to late 30's. Whilst I do not believe any direct prior relationship existed between any of the victims and the offender I believe the offender is familiar with, in some capacity, XX college. I believe the offender will most likely be in some form of white collar employment and...............

==//==

[14] In assessing the spatial patterns relative to these offenses I have annexed a map of what I consider to be locations of relevance concerning these crimes and this appears as Appendix (A). You will note that I have taken a range of measurements and illustrated this by the use of circles on the map attached. Based upon these measurements you will observe that the suburbs of Reading and Lynn have been identified ....

Box 11.5. Evaluation.

tion. In broad terms, and as briefly mentioned in the previous chapter, investigative suggestions may be of a proactive or reactive nature. Proactive suggestions or tactics are those that, for example, may assist the investigation in the generation of new leads or strategies that may prevent or inhibit the commission of further offenses or indeed lead to an opportunity to apprehend the offender. Reactive suggestions are predominantly those pertaining more to information or events that are already available to the investigation, such as the prioritization of further inquiries for an established list of suspects or locations for investigation.

It may prove useful in the investigative application(s) section to adopt subheadings of proactive and reactive for ease of reference. Within each of these subheadings, separate dot points can be presented individually describing each proffered suggestion. Consequently, in contrast to the flowing narrative of the evaluation, the information canvassed in the investigative application(s) section may be systematically subdivided into smaller dot point segments. Each of these dot points or subsections should then contain an outline of the relevant information for specific investigative application. A limited example of an investigative suggestion section appears in Box 11.6.

Step 7: Specified Questions

One section that may also be included in a report is a questions and answers section. Obviously, such a section is not relevant if the consulting organization to the matter has not elected to raise any specific questions regarding the matter with the consultant. In the event that no specific ques-

[15] Investigative Applications

Based upon my evaluation of the individual most likely to have committed these murders I offer the following suggestions which can, at your discretion, be adopted by your investigation to assist in apprehending this individual. I have labeled these suggestions as being either of a proactive or reactive nature:

Proactive Tactics

- Attempt arrest via undercover decoys

[16] There is some suggestion owing to the physical characteristics of the murdered women that in selecting victims the offender is operating on some generic archetype. Some of these discernible commonalties include women who are youthful in appearance with long blond hair who were wearing dresses at the time of their attack. It is also apparent that the offender demonstrates a seasonal pattern in the commission of these offenses. Furthermore, all attacks have transpired in the XXXXXX area between the hours of XXXXpm and XXXXpm. Based upon the combination of these factors one possibility which could be explored is the concentrated patrolling of……..

- ………..
- ………..

Reactive Tactics

- Suspect Prioritization – XXXX College Connection

[17] A number of factors surrounding these crimes as detailed in the case summary suggest that the offender possesses some connection with or knowledge of XXXX college. Some of these factors are that all victims have been students at XXXX college, all were last seen departing the XXXX college and all victims were evidently attacked during the XXXXX break when the campus population is reduced and therefore potential witnesses minimized. Based upon these factors I would recommend carefully researching the backgrounds of all established suspects to examine whether any possess some form of link to XXXX College. It may not be that the offender has any obvious association with XXXX college like, for example, being formerly enrolled there as a student, but may be more of an indirect association such as performing seasonal, casual work for the college, having a sibling who attends the college, or making odd deliveries to the campus etc. Questioning of suspects to explore any connection with the college may prove useful in……………..

- …………

Box 11.6. Investigative application(s).

tions are asked, as a professional matter it is nonetheless wise to include a "Specified Questions" heading followed by a short statement to the effect that none were posed to you.

In most instances, however, investigators seeking a criminal profile formulate a number of specific questions they expect the consultant to answer as best he or she can. There are a number of important factors to bear in mind when including such a section in the report. First, and most fundamentally, a response should always be provided to every question that is raised irrespective of the level of formality or perceived relevance or otherwise of the question. Under no circumstance should any question be ignored and thus not included in the report. In answering questions, responses should be focused and directly relate to the issue(s) raised. Responses should, wherever possible, also include a readily comprehensible explanation outlining the rationale for each response. Incumbent to such an explanation should be references to items of information within the report that support or inform the response. These procedures are advocated to once again promote transparency and thus professionalism in the preparation of the report. It should therefore be apparent that yes or no answers are rarely suitable. If, for example, a yes/no response is specifically requested, it should be provided followed with an explanation as to why this particular response is offered. Finally, it is important to readily admit to limitations concerning a provided opinion. If an appropriate answer is simply not known, this should be honestly stated. Similarly, should a question require a response that involves a significant deviation from the consultant profiler's domain of knowledge and/or expertise, a clear statement acknowledging this circumstance should also be made. Similarly, should a response necessitate a substantial degree of qualification or speculation, this should also be clearly indicated.

The format of any questions section should be simple and clear. Each question should be listed in the form of a subheading. The question should, wherever possible, be reproduced exactly as posed. Consequently, questions should not be paraphrased or amended in any manner, but rather repeated verbatim. Similarly, the chronology of questions should follow the order in which they were posed and each should therefore be numbered accordingly. If, for example, several questions have been posed, some of which occur in a subsequent communication to the date when the original consultation was commissioned, the chronology of these questions should also include the specific dates of when any subsequent questions were raised. Once again, a limited hypothetical example of a specified questions section appears in Box 11.7.

Step 8: Concluding Statements

It is strongly recommended that any report finish with a concluding statement that indicates the author's availability and preparedness to assist fur-

Specified Questions

[25] I will now in turn provide a response to each of the specific questions raised in your letter to me of XX/XX/XXXX and in my two subsequent telephone conversations with XXXX of your organization on XX/XX/XXXX and XX/XX/XXXX.

[26] (1) *What is the likelihood that this series of murders will continue?*

It is my belief that the offender is a serial sexual killer who is unlikely to voluntarily desist in the commission of further offenses. Naturally, a number of intervening factors may account for a perceived cessation in activity such as sickness, death, incarceration for another offense etc. However, allowing for such mitigating factors to be discounted, I suspect further murders are likely to occur unless the offender is apprehended. I provide this answer based upon a variety of behavioral factors (see Kocsis & Irwin, 1998) demonstrated in the commission of three previous murders which are characteristic of sexual murderers. These behavioral factors include……………………
………………………………..
………………………………...

[27] (1) *What is the likelihood that the offender will respond to the public announcement?*

I think it quite unlikely that the offender will……………..

Box 11.7. Specified questions.

ther. Some offer should be made to elaborate on or clarify any issue should this be required. Readers should be encouraged to contact you as the author if they so wish. Furthermore, it should be emphasized that the information contained in the report is contemporaneous with the time of consultation and the material made available for consideration at that time; hence, any further material that may come to hand may assist in adjusting, focusing, and possibly strengthening the information which is the subject of the criminal profile.

Furthermore, in the conclusion the report should also include a statement to the effect that the consultant profiler has read and is familiar with the relevant code of ethical practice concerning expert consultants. Naturally, these codes will vary from jurisdiction to jurisdiction so the reference details of the code by which the consultant is affirming their readiness to be bound should be accurately identified. Good ethical practice also dictates that a copy of the consulting profiler's curriculum vitae (CV) be attached for the reader's information and reference. The purpose of attaching a CV is to once again demonstrate transparency in providing the reader with some information concerning the nature of the consultant profiler's expertise and credentials. Finally, as a professional courtesy, the report should conclude with a statement again thanking the organization for electing to consult you, the profiler. A simple example of a concluding statement is provided in Box 11.8.

Specified Questions

[25] I will now in turn provide a response to each of the specific questions raised in your letter to me of XX/XX/XXXX and in my two subsequent telephone conversations with XXXX of your organization on XX/XX/XXXX and XX/XX/XXXX.

[26] *(1) What is the likelihood that this series of murders will continue?*

It is my belief that the offender is a serial sexual killer who is unlikely to voluntarily desist in the commission of further offenses. Naturally, a number of intervening factors may account for a perceived cessation in activity such as sickness, death, incarceration for another offense etc. However, allowing for such mitigating factors to be discounted, I suspect further murders are likely to occur unless the offender is apprehended. I provide this answer based upon a variety of behavioral factors (see Kocsis & Irwin, 1998) demonstrated in the commission of three previous murders which are characteristic of sexual murderers. These behavioral factors include……………………
………………………………
………………………………

[27] *(2) What is the likelihood that the offender will respond to the public announcement?*

I think it quite unlikely that the offender will………………

==//==

Conclusions

[35] I wish to again thank you for your decision in electing to consult me on this matter. Please note that the conclusions drawn in this report are based upon my best attempts to evaluate the information that has been made available to me at this juncture. Naturally should further information become available further refinement of the profile may be required depending of course upon the nature of this material. Finally, I wish to advise that I have read and agree to abide by the XXXXXXX XXXXXXX code of professional ethics and have attached a copy of my current CV for your information and reference.

Should you require elaboration, clarification or have any further questions pertaining to this report, please do not hesitate to contact me on XXXXXX.

Yours faithfully,

Richard N. Kocsis Ph.D.

Box 11.8. Concluding statements. The concluding statements appear in larger font.

Step 9: References and Appendices

All reports should, if necessary, attach a separate reference list and any appendix referred to in the report. The number of appendices is purely dependent on the material and issues covered in the report. One clear example of an appendix should be any mentioned map that was used in the development of a geographic profile as referred to earlier. Another suitable item for the appendix may be any particular research article pertinent to the criminal profile. This may only, for example, consist of a few photocopied pages from a book or may include an entire academic article.

The presentation and format of a reference list and any appendices are entirely open to the consultant's preference. Thus, no particular method for citation and referencing is recommended, only that appropriate sources are indeed cited with an adjoining reference list compiled at the end of the report. Similarly, no particular style of formatting is advocated for the creation of any appendices.

Conclusion

The material canvassed throughout this chapter aims to serve as a guide for various conventions that should be observed when compiling a written criminal profile. The extent to which these suggestions should be adhered to will naturally depend on the circumstances of the matter and the nature of the report/profile requested. The principles underlying the various format recommendations canvassed throughout this chapter have been developed to promote transparency, accountability, and professionalism in the composition of a criminal profile. In some instances, some of the detailed conventions may not be possible to follow and this circumstance does not connotate impropriety on the part of the profiler. However, it should be recognized that such circumstances represent a departure from the conventions described herein. Professional credibility is maximized when opportunity for independent scrutiny and assessment is possible. Indeed, this principle underscores many disciplines and its practitioners: the publication of research in anonymously peer-reviewed journals is but only one example of this. Consequently, the principles described in this chapter strive to achieve a standard of professionalism in developing a criminal profile.

Epilogue

Fighting Fire With Fire

One conundrum I have often contemplated is why the scientific development of criminal profiling has been so slow. In promoting criminal profiling while concurrently excusing any potential failings, authors dating back as far as the early 1980s have described the development of profiling as being in its infancy *(1,2)*. Approximately 25 years later, authors still appear to be referring to the embryonic state of profiling *(3)*. As Oleson *(4)* poignantly observed, it is long past time that criminal profiling grew up!

Within most scholarly disciplines a process of attrition characterizes progress in the sense that newer, better concepts emerge to replace older ones. In this context, some consideration needs to be given as to why some concepts in the area of criminal profiling have enjoyed such remarkable longevity. The material discussed throughout this book should dispel any naïve notions concerning the adequacy of previous work and research in the area. However, this state of affairs I believe is not because of any single reason, but is instead, best explained by a range of factors in combination.

Probably the most frustrating is the transposition of popular culture depictions concerning the robustness of the criminal profiling technique onto some of its real world equivalents. Cinema, television, and true crime literature abounds with romanticized depictions of heroic profilers who ingeniously and unfailingly solve crimes *(5–7)*. Such favorable, albeit fanciful, depictions in my view frequently promote unrealistic impressions concerning the credibility of profilers, the techniques they advocate, and their affiliated organizations *(8)*. Regrettably, all of my studies combined cannot compete with the promotional impact of what can be conveyed by a single Hollywood blockbuster movie.

From: *Criminal Profiling: Principles and Practice*
By: R. N. Kocsis © Humana Press Inc., Totowa, NJ

Another factor I believe to be central to the tardy scientific development of profiling involves access to data. In this modern age, the slow development of criminal profiling cannot be attributed to a shortage of suitably qualified individuals throughout the world prepared to develop the technique. Instead, I believe a significant mitigating factor is the hurdle encountered when attempting to access data to undertake research. From my own experiences, somewhat peculiar and quite arbitrary restrictions concerning the confidentiality of data such as closed case materials *(9)* are often imposed on external researchers by the custodians of such data. The vagaries of these restrictions are frequently overlooked. In many cases, useful material has already been aired in the public domain in the form of court hearings. Confronted by such obstacles, it can easily be seen how this circumstance stifles researchers in the production of new research.

A third factor integral to the slow development of profiling is the very environment within which it is often applied—namely policing organizations. Legal and criminological scholars have long observed the often authoritarian and acutely insular nature of the organizational culture found to prevail in policing organizations *(10–14)*. Such an environment is unlikely to be conducive to the unfettered testing of theories that more routinely characterize scientific disciplines. Instead, unwarranted distrust and even the arbitrary dismissal of individuals who are perceived to be external to the policing community is often encountered. Indeed, research contributions even when made may be unfairly devalued or ignored altogether on the basis of its production by an outsider. To compound these problems, something of an industry has evolved within many policing organizations concerning the practice of criminal profiling *(15,16)*. Training and accreditation programs for profiling appear to be more concerned with the promotion of personnel within police organizations *(17,18)* rather than on the impartial evaluation and development of the technique. Consequently, it is difficult to gauge to what extent, if at all, rivaling research and theories would genuinely be embraced were they not to unreservedly endorse the practices of those with their own vocational interests in profiling *(19)*.

Unquestionably, the most disheartening factor surrounding the development of criminal profiling involves the misconception by some that scientifically grounded progress is in fact being made. In my view, this problem, to some extent, stems from the lack of unified regulation surrounding the practice of criminal profiling *(19)*. Credentials vary dramatically among individuals who offer profiling services and readily promote their expertise in this area *(19)*. Consequently, there exists what can euphemistically be described as blissful ignorance of the scientific method and the conventions for the production of scientifically vetted (i.e., valid) research. Despite the sincerest of intentions to aid in the investigation of crime, the coining of new terms and phrases combined with sprinklings of previous criminological literature and anecdotal experiences often dominate the profiling landscape and are mistakenly confused as constituting original, empirical, and scientifically robust research in and of itself *(20)*.

The various factors raised thus far are largely beyond my influence, however, there is one within my sphere and I conclude by discussing it. As previously indicated, it is necessary when considering the comparatively tardy development of criminal profiling to consider why some profiling concepts display such remarkable longevity in light of more recent research that highlight limitations. Ironically, I believe the explanation for this circumstance lies not in the brilliance of these older concepts, but rather, their simplicity in terms of comprehension. One example of this phenomenon is the organized/disorganized dichotomy, which arguably represents the cornerstone piece of research underlying the approach to profiling espoused by the FBI and referred to as Criminal Investigative Analysis *(21,22)*. Despite many researchers having highlighted the limitations of this dichotomy *(23–25)*, it is research that still seems to enjoy currency. It is my view, however, that the appeal of this dichotomy and the approach to profiling advocated comes from its easy comprehension in comparison to often more technical literature. Statistical research methodologies such as multidimensional scaling are, admittedly, neither common nor easy-to-follow procedures even among statisticians and social scientists. With a loss of comprehension, arguably, even the most compelling reasoning is likely to fail when contrasted with a simpler, more palatable concept.

Personnel of law enforcement agencies throughout the world are seldom imbued with the luxury of time to learn and thus fully appreciate the intricacies of complex research methodologies and statistical procedures. Instead, their focus is, understandably, more often on the pragmatic application of readily tangible concepts. A concept that is not fully comprehended is, quite justifiably, unlikely to be adopted. In this regard, the greatest weakness of my own research endeavors over the years is its complexity that may in turn impede its comprehension and broader application. I have resolved that now is the time to fight fire with fire. In effect, if the strengths and benefits of the Crime Action Profiling research are to be truly appreciated, then the comprehension of its principles must, wherever possible, be refashioned in a more user-friendly manner to allow for a greater number of people to understand and apply them in a practical manner. By striving to improve the comprehension of the Crime Action Profiling research through the pages of this book, I hope to also highlight the work that still needs to be done to genuinely progress the development of criminal profiling.

References

1. Rossi, D. (1982). Crime scene behavioral analysis: Another tool for the law enforcement investigator. Police Chief, 18(4),152–155.
2. Vorpagel, R.E. (1982). Painting psychological profiles: Charlatanism, coincidence, charisma or new science. Police Chief, 3(8), 156–159.
3. McCrary, G. and Ramsland, K. (2003). The unknown darkness. New York: Morrow.
4. Oleson, J.C. (1996). Psychological profiling: Does it actually work? Forensic Update, 46, 11–14.
5. Harris, T. (1985). The red dragon. New York: Heineman.
6. Harris, T. (1989). The silence of the lambs. New York: Heineman.
7. Harris, T. (1999). Hannibal. New York: Heineman.
8. Muller, D.A. (2000). Criminal profiling: real science or just wishful thinking? Homicide Studies, 4(3), 234–264.
9. Kocsis, R.N. and Coleman, S. (2000). The unexplored ethics of criminal psychological profiling. In: Godwin, M.G., ed. Criminal psychology and forensic technology: A collaborative approach to effective profiling. New York: CRC Press, pp. 323–338.
10. Reiner, R. (1985). The politics of the police. UK: Wheatsheaf Books.
11. Reiner, R. (1992). The politics of the police, 2nd ed. UK: Harvester & Wheatsheaf.
12. Reiner, R. (2000). The politics of the police, 3rd ed. UK: Oxford University Press.
13. Reiner, R. (1996). Policing, vol. I. Dartmouth: Aldershot.
14. Reiner, R. (1996). Policing, vol. II. Dartmouth: Aldershot.
15. Douglas, J.E. and Olshaker, M. (1995). Mindhunter. New York: Scribner.
16. Wilson, C. and Seaman, D. (1992). The serial killers. London: Cox & Wyman.
17. Beck, J.P., O'Sullivan, B.J., Ogilvie, A.B. (1989). An Australian violent criminal apprehension programme: A feasibility study. Adelaide: National Police Research Unit.
18. Rayment, M. (1995). Inside the mind of a criminal. NSW Police News, 75, 15–18.
19. Kocsis, R. N. and Palermo, G.B. (2005). Ten major problems with criminal profiling. American Journal of Forensic Psychiatry, 26(2), 45–67.
20. Palermo, G.B. and Kocsis, R.N. (2005). Offender profiling: An introduction to the sociopsychological analysis of violent crime. Springfield, IL: CC Thomas.
21. Ressler, R.K., Burgess, A.W., Douglas, J.E., Hartman, C.R., D'Agostino, R.B. (1986). Sexual killers and their victims: Identifying patterns through crime scene analysis. Journal of Interpersonal Violence, 1, 288–308.
22. Douglas, J.E., Burgess, A.W., Burgess, A.G., Ressler, R.K. (1992). Crime classification manual. New York: Simon & Schuster.
23. Godwin, G.M. (2000). Hunting serial predators. New York: CRC Press.
24. Canter, D. (1994). Criminal shadows. London: HarperCollins.

25. Kocsis, R.N., Irwin, H.J., Hayes, A.F. (1998). Organised and disorganised behaviour syndromes in arsonists: A validation study of a psychological profiling concept. Psychiatry, Psychology and Law, 5, 117–130.

Appendix A

Understanding Descriptive and Inferential Statistics

A Beginner's Guide

The Scientific Method, Measurement, and Descriptive Statistics

All disciplines concerned with the scientific examination of any topic rely on the observation and systematic measurement of some phenomenon. From these measurements, explanations or theories are proposed to account for such measurements. Also through the use of measurement comes the investigation of theories by the creation of tests or experiments that pose hypotheses. Invariably, a hypothesis is made concerning a particular issue and then the observed outcomes derived from the constructed experiment are measured as a way of evaluating the validity of a given hypothesis. The theory is supported when the measured outcome concords with the predictions, and refuted when it does not.

Chapters 2–4 describe a series of experiments that investigate various issues related to the composition and accuracy of criminal profiles. All of these studies were accomplished by undertaking various measurements of particular aspects of a criminal profile and evaluating what, if anything, those measurements suggested, and whether or not they concord with any given theory or hypothesis. One crucial issue in understanding these experiments is being able to follow how any observed and measured outcomes (i.e., the results) are interpreted as either supporting or rejecting the hypothesis of the experiment. Rather than relying on arbitrary and personal views, the scientific method

From: *Criminal Profiling: Principles and Practice*
By: R. N. Kocsis © Humana Press Inc., Totowa, NJ

typically relies on statistics to impartially inform these decisions. With the aid of statistics, calculations can be made in respect of any measurements taken on any subject matter, that in statistical parlance are referred to as data. Similarly, any given calculation and interpretation of results in respect of data are typically referred to as statistical analysis.

Broadly speaking, and as far as this introductory guide is concerned, there are two forms of statistical analysis: descriptive and inferential. As their names suggest, these two types of statistics are used for either the purposes of description or inference. As will hopefully become apparent, these two types of statistical analysis complement each other. That is, descriptive statistics often provide an initial description of the measured phenomena in question, whereas the more sophisticated inferential statistics allow for the inference or determination of any posed question or hypothesis.

As a very rudimentary demonstration of the empirical procedures involved with scientific research as well as the operation and differences between descriptive and inferential statistics, a simple hypothetical example will be used by way of illustration involving a farmer who owns two different apple-peeling machines. The farmer would like to determine how many apples machines A and B can each peel in 1 hour. To answer this question, the farmer decides to undertake a test that, in fact, represents a simple experiment. He inserts an equal number of apples into both machines and then times (i.e., measures) them for 1 hour to see how many apples they respectively peel. This process of counting the number of peeled apples within 1 hour relies on observation and measurement. From this first trial the farmer notes that machine A peeled 9 apples and machine B peeled 14 apples. These two values of 9 and 14 now represent data that is relevant to the issue of how many apples the two machines can each peel.

Another important component to the scientific method is concerned with repetition and more importantly recognition of the reliability of measurements being affected by random events or chance. For example, for the farmer to be satisfied that machine A consistently peels 9 apples and machine B consistently peels 14 apples he may wish to repeat the experiment to see how reliable this initial measurement regarding the performance of the two machines is. Perhaps, during the first trial machine A encountered one apple that was particularly difficult to peel and this actually slowed the process down considerably from its usual pace in peeling apples. Alternatively, perhaps machine B by coincidence had apples that were exceptionally easy to peel and hence it was able to peel more apples than usual. To discount such possibilities that might undermine the reliability of the farmer's measurements, two further trials of counting and thereby measuring the number of apples machines A and B can each respectively peel is undertaken. Following the conclusion of these two trials the farmer observes and records that machine A peeled 10 apples on its second trial and 11 apples on its third trial. Concurrently, machine B peeled 16 apples on its second trial and 15 apples on its third trial. The collection of these measurements (i.e., data) represents a sample pertaining to the relative performance of the two machines in peeling apples. The farmer has now recorded measurements that indicate that within 1 hour, machine A was capable of peeling 9, 10, and 11 apples, respectively, whereas machine B peeled 14, 16, and 15 apples. The farmer now has a number of measurements relative to the capabilities of his two machines, however, he now needs to determine how many apples each machine typically peels within 1 hour.

Up until this point we have considered the systematic procedures of observation and measurement that are integral to the scientific method. However, to answer the question of how many apples each machine can typically peel now requires the use of statistics and, specifically, descriptive statistics to describe the typical number of peeled apples. This is accomplished by assessing the average number of apples peeled by machines A and B respectively in repeated trials. This average is referred to as the mean. The mean is calculated by taking the sum total of all data and dividing it by the number of trials. Thus, the calculations of the mean for machine A is the sum of all the number of apples peeled in each experiment (the data) divided by the number of trials conducted (i.e., [9 + 10 + 11] divided by 3—that is, 30 divided by 3). By adopting this procedure, machine A has a mean value of 10, whereas machine B has a mean of 15. By following the scientific method of conducting three separate empirical trials and measuring the number of apples peeled by each machine for each trial, and with the aid of the descriptive statistic known as the mean, the farmer can determine that within 1 hour machine A typically peels 10 apples, whereas machine B typically peels 15.

Inferential Statistics: Whether Differences Are More Than Chance Occurrence

The hypothetical example of the farmer with the apple-peeling machine should have demonstrated the importance of observation and measurement in forming the empirical basis of scientific research. This example has been used to highlight in simple terms the use of a descriptive statistic in providing an indication of how many apples each of the machines typically peeled based on the data derived from the three separate trials conducted. Having ascertained the mean number of apples that each machine can peel, it then becomes important to question whether the difference in the mean number of apples peeled between the two machines is reliable or, in statistical parlance, statistically significant.

In a purely descriptive context it can already be stated that the mean value of 15 for machine B is higher than the mean value of 10 for machine A. However, it must be recognized that although 10 and 15 may seem like obvious differences, scientific research is often confronted by far more difficult conundrums. Many studies often deal with vast numbers derived from differing samples. When dealing with such large samples the numbers may not be as easily distinguishable. For example, the difference between a mean score of 12.46 and another of 11.99 may not seem too large. However, if these two values derived from samples of several hundred thousand individual measurements, then the higher value of 12.46 could indeed prove to be a very important difference. Additionally, the discipline of science is acutely aware of the generally capricious nature of the world and the real possibility of chance influencing occurrences. Consequently, it becomes necessary to assess whether the observed measurements from the three trials conducted by the farmer and the mean values derived from them are merely artifacts of chance or whether there really was a difference in the performance of the two machines.

Inferential statistics may be used to gauge the reliable probability of any given measurement. That is, inferential statistics are primarily concerned with ascertaining the probability of a series of observed and recorded measurements being due to chance under some previously specified hypothesis. Therefore, in our case, inferential statistics are a tool for determining whether the two mean values are different enough for us to believe that the measurements cannot be dismissed as occurring purely due to chance.

There are numerous types of inferential statistics that rely on differing formulas with varying levels of sophistication for their calculation. Two common forms of inferential statistics involve the use of *t*-tests and analysis of variance (ANOVA). The calculations for these statistics are discussed in depth in many textbooks on statistics. For the purpose of this book, however, it is important to simply understand the functions of such statistical tests. That is, these tests represent statistical methods for calculating by way of mathematical formulae the probability of a result occurring because of chance. Returning to our apple-peeling machine example, inferential statistical analysis can calculate the p or probability value. The discipline of statistics has a specific procedure to determine how this p value may be interpreted by indexing it with a conceptual standard that is referred to as an α level. The most common α level is typically a mathematical value of 0.05. Consequently, if a p value is determined to be below the threshold of 0.05 then the conclusion is that the values are indeed statistically significant. However, if the calculated value is above the α level, then it is not statistically significant and thus there exists some possibility that chance may account for the measured values. There is some debate as to what is the acceptable α level and this is very much dependent on the standard sought. Effectively, the lower the α level, the more conservative the standard and vice versa. Returning to the example of the apple-peeling machine, by the use of inferential statistical analysis it can be determined that the mean values for each machine are indeed statistically significant. That is, Box 1 indicates a *p* value of 0.0036. Because 0.0036 is well less than the chosen α value of 0.05, it can be stated that the mean values of 10 and 15 are indeed different. In interpreting this result, it can be concluded that the efficiency of machine B surpasses that of machine A by way of a statistically significant margin. That is, machine B does indeed peel more apples than machine A and this result is unlikely to result from any random chance event.

To understand inferential statistical analysis it is also important to clearly note that results can be found that are not statistically significant. For example, returning once again to our apple-peeling machines, imagine that the calculated *p* value was not 0.0036 but instead, for arguments sake, 0.07. In this circumstance, when using the α level of 0.05 we would interpret the calculation as not being statistically significant. That is, 0.07 is more than the α level of 0.05. When interpreting this result in the context of the apple-peeling machines we would then say although machine A attained a mean value of 10 and machine B attained a mean value of 15, the margin of difference between these two values was not found to be statistically significant. That is, although we can descriptively observe a difference between these two mean values, we cannot discount the possibility that this margin of difference between the two mean values as possibly being attributable to a chance event when adopting an α value of 0.05.

Finally, as previously mentioned, the chosen standard in determining these α levels can vary. The most commonly adopted α level is 0.05. However, in some circumstances an extremely low α level may be chosen such as, for example, 0.0001 (which is incredibly low) or alternatively, a high α level such as 0.10 (which is not as conservative). The advantages and disadvantages of using varying α levels are an issue totally based on their relativity in interpreting the derived *p* values. For example, if an α level of 0.0001 was adopted with our apple-peeling machines then none of the *p* values previously discussed would be considered statistically significant. However, it could be argued that an α level of 0.0001 is ridiculously stringent and that in most reasonable instances a *p* value of 0.0036 would indeed constitute a statistically significant result. The reverse of this argument is also applicable. Thus, if an α level of 0.10 was utilized then all of the previously mentioned *p* values

Descriptive Statistic

	Machine (A)	Machine (B)
Trial 1	9	14
Trial 2	10	16
Trial 3	11	15
	Mean = 10	Mean = 15

The above Table shows the 'mean' calculated for each machine over 3 separate trials. Consequently, the mean or average number of apples peeled by machine (A) is 10, and for machine (B) it is 15. Thus, based on the data derived from each of the three trials machine (A) typically peels 10 apples while machine (B) typically peels 15.

Inferential Statistics

Having established that the typical number of apples peeled by machine (A) and (B) is 10 and 15 respectively, is it reasonable to conclude that the number of apples peeled by each machine is a reliable result? In a "descriptive" context we can say that the values of 10 and 15 are different and that a trend is apparent with machine (B) peeling more apples. However, inferential statistics may be used to discount the possibility of chance accounting for these different results.

	Machine (A)		Machine (B)	
Mean values for each machine	10	vs	15	P-value 0.0036

Alpha level set at 0.05:
A P value found to be below this is statistically significant whilst a value above 0.05 is not.

The data is calculated using an inferential statistic and obtains a P value of 0.0036. As this value is below the alpha level this indicates that the difference between 10 and 15 is 'statistically significant' and is unlikely therefore to be attributable to chance. With the use of inferential statistics it can be concluded with more confidence that the values of 10 and 15 are indeed different. That is, machine (B) does indeed peel more apples in comparison to machine (A). Furthermore, we could conclude this to be more probably than not the case each time the same trial is conducted for each machine as we can be confident that some chance event has not influenced the respective results for each machine.

Box 1

would be considered statistically significant including a *p* value of 0.07. However, in this circumstance the amount of confidence we could attribute to these findings as not being accounted for by chance would not be as great as if we were to use the α level of 0.05. Thus, the use of α levels in interpreting the *p* values is a matter of relative standards.

ACKNOWLEDGMENT

The author acknowledges with gratitude the assistance of Jenny Middledorp, Department of Statistics, MacQuarie University, for her review of this appendix.

Appendix B

Labels and Definitions for All Variables in Chapter 7

Serial Rape CAP Model

Variable group	Variable label	Definition (category labels and coding; numbers in parentheses indicated categories combined in the code)
Victim characteristics	VSEX	Victim's sex (male = 0; female = 1)
	VAGE	Victim's age (20 years old or less= 0; 21 years or older = 1)
	VTRANSPT	Victim's usual mode of transport (self-modes [1, 2, 4] = 0; relies on others [3, 5, 6, 7] = 1)
	VMARITAL	Victim's marital status (single/ex-partner [1, 3, 4, 5, 6] = 0; partnered [2] = 1)
	VLIVEWTH	Victim living with (alone [8] = 0; others [1–7] = 1)
	VINCAPAC	Victim incapacitated at time of initial contact (no = 0; yes = 1)
Offender characteristics	ORACE	Offender's race (white = 0; non-white = 1)
	OAGE	Offender's age (20 years old or less = 0; 21 years or older = 1)
	OLANG	Offender's language background (monolingual = 0; bilingual = 1)
	OHEIGHT	Offender's height (short = 0; medium, tall = 1)
	OWEIGHT	Offender's weight (lighter = 0; heavier = 1)
	OBUILD	Offender's build (small = 0; medium, large = 1)
	OHAIRSHA	Offender's hair shade (lighter = 0; darker = 1)

(*continued on next page*)

Variable group	Variable label	Definition (category labels and coding; numbers in parentheses indicated categories combined in the code)
	OHAIRLEN	Offender's hair length (short/none [1–3] = 0; medium/long [4–6] =1)
	OHAIRSTY	Offender's hair style (neat/tidy = 0; unkempt = 1)
	OHAIRCOL	Offender's hair color (red, gray, or white = 0; brown or black = 1)
	OEYECOL	Offender's eye color (light eyes = 0; dark eyes = 1)
	OTEETH	Offender's teeth (not noticed = 0; noticeably imperfect = 1)
	OFACHAIR	Offender had facial hair (no = 0; yes = 1)
	OSCAR	Offender had scars/marks (no = 0; yes = 1)
	OOUTFEAT	Offender had outstanding physical features (no = 0; yes = 1)
	OACCENT	Offender had an accent (no = 0; yes = 1)
	OMENTILL	Offender showed evidence of mental illness (no = 0; yes = 1)
	OODOURS	Offender had noticeable odor (no = 0; yes = 1)
	ODRUGALC	Offender showed evidence of drug/alcohol use (no = 0; yes = 1)
	OINTERST	Offender visited interstate in past 10 years (no = 0; yes = 1)
	OINTERNA	Offender lived/visited internationally over past 10 years (no = 0; yes = 1)
	OMARITAL	Offender's marital status (single/ex-partner [1, 3, 4, 5] = 0; partnered [2] = 1)
	OLIVEWTH	Offender living with (alone [8] = 0; others [1–7] = 1)
	OJOBTYPE	Offender job type (unemployed = 0; employed = 1)
	OLIFESTY	Offender's general lifestyle (non-criminal [1, 2, 4, 8, 11–13] = 0; criminal [3, 5–7, 9–10] = 1)
	OCRIMST	Offender's criminal status (non-offender = 0; statutory release = 1)
	OSEXHAB	Offender's sexual habits (heterosexual = 0; homosexual/bisexual = 1)
	OMENPROB	Offender displayed symptoms or had been treated for mental problems (no = 0; yes = 1)
	OPOSPROP	Offender possessed other's property (no = 0; yes = 1)
	OCONFESS	Offender admitted to other similar crimes of violence (no = 0; yes = 1)

(*continued on next page*)

Variable group	Variable label	Definition (category labels and coding; numbers in parentheses indicated categories combined in the code)
	OVEHUSED	Offender used a vehicle in this incident (no = 0; yes = 1)
	OVEHSTAT	Offender's vehicle status (owned = 0; not owned = 1)
	OVEHTYPE	Offender's vehicle type (car = 0; van/SUV/truck = 1)
Offender–victim interaction characteristics	INEIGHBR	Neighborhood initial contact (residential = 0; non-residential = 1)
	IPRIORAC	Prior activity initial contact area (no = 0; yes = 1)
	IPOTWITN	Potential witnesses at initial contact area (no = 0; yes = 1)
	ICONTACT	Location of initial contact scene (indoors = 0; outdoors = 1)
	ILIVQUAR	Initial contact: living quarters (no = 0; yes = 1)
	IPUBPLAC	Initial contact: public place (no = 0; yes = 1)
	IOUTDOOR	Initial contact: outdoors (no = 0; yes = 1)
	IFAMSITE	Offender's familiarity with initial contact site (familiar = 0; unfamiliar = 1)
	IVCLOTH	Victim's clothing at initial contact site (nothing done [1] = 0; something done [2–5] = 1)
	CISAME	Initial contact site same as crime site (no = 0; yes = 1)
	CINOUT	Crime site was indoors or outdoors (indoors = 0; outdoors = 1)
	CCOMMUM	Crime scene community type (city [2,3] = 0; non-city [1, 4, 5] = 1)
	CLIVQUAR	Crime scene: living quarters (no = 0; yes = 1)
	CPUBPLAC	Crime scene: public place (no = 0; yes = 1)
	COUTDOOR	Crime scene: outdoors (no = 0; yes = 1)
	CFAMSITE	Offender's familiarity with crime scene (familiar = 0; unfamiliar = 1)
	CFINCONT	How did victim/offender contact end (released = 0; escaped/interruption = 1)
	RISAME	Recovery site same as initial contact site (no = 0; yes = 1)
	RCSAME	Recovery site same as crime scene (no = 0; yes = 1)
	RCOMMUN	Recovery site community type (city [2, 3] = 0; non-city [1,4,5] = 1)

(*continued on next page*)

Variable group	Variable label	Definition (category labels and coding; numbers in parentheses indicated categories combined in the code)
	RLIVQUAR	Recovery scene: living quarters (no = 0; yes = 1)
	ROUTDOOR	Recovery scene: outdoors (no = 0; yes = 1)
	RFAMSITE	Offender's familiarity with recovery site (familiar = 0; unfamiliar = 1)
Crime scene characteristics	OVSELECT	Offender's selection of the victim (opportunistic = 0; planned = 1 [*Plan attack*])
	OVCON	Offender approached victim with a con (no = 0; yes = 1 [*O con V*])
	OVSURPR	Offender approached victim by surprise (no = 0; yes = 1 [*O surprise V*])
	OVBLITZ	Offender approached victim with a blitz attack (no = 0; yes = 1 [*O blitz V*])
	VACTOAPP	Victim's activities when offender approached (home = 0; public = 1 [*V act O app*])
	OFORCUSE	How much force offender used (enough to control = 0; excessive = 1 [*Excess force*])
	FORCEBEF	Force was used before sex (no = 0; yes = 1 [*Force bf sex*])
	FORCERES	Force used when victim resisted (no = 0; yes = 1 [*Force resist*])
	FORCEDUR	Force was used during sex (no = 0; yes = 1 [*Force dg sex*])
	VINJURED	Extent of victim's injuries (none = 0; some injuries suffered = 1 [*V injured*])
	OANGER	Extent of offender anger evident (none/some = 0; extreme = 1 [*Anger extrem*])
	VICRESIS	Victim offered resistance (no resistance = 0; some resistance = 1 [*V resisted*])
	REACTRES	Reaction to victim resistance (ignore/back down = 0; threaten/force = 1 [*O threaten*])
	SEXACTV	Evidence of sex act with victim (no = 0; yes = 1 [*Sex with V*])
	SEXASSAU	Nature of sexual assault (assaulted internally = 0; assaulted externally = 1 [*External sex*])
	SEMENBOD	Semen found in body cavities of victim (no = 0; yes = 1 [*Semen in bod*])
	OSEXDYSF	Evidence of offender sex dysfunction (no = 0; yes = 1 [*O sex dysfun*])
	OOVERDYS	Offender did something to overcome sexual dysfunction (no = 0; yes = 1 [*O ov sex dys*])

(*continued on next page*)

Variable group	Variable label	Definition (category labels and coding; numbers in parentheses indicated categories combined in the code)
	ATCHFEAR	Offender attitude toward victim became fearful/ apologetic (no = 0; yes = 1 [*O more Fear*])
	ATCHANGR	Offender attitude toward victim became more angry (no = 0; yes = 1 [*O more Angry*])
	OVTALK	Offender required victim to talk (no = 0; yes = 1 [*O req V talk*])
	OTALKSLF	Offender talked about himself to victim (no = 0; yes = 1 [*O talk abt O*])
	OQUESTV	Offender questioned victim about personal life (no = 0; yes = 1 [*O question V*])
	OIMAGEV	Offender image projected to victim (neutral = 0; managed (1, 3) = 1 [*O manip imag*])
	ODEMEANV	Offender demeanour to victim (neutral = 0; managed (1, 3) = 1 [*O manip beh*])
	VONEGOT	Negotiation between victim and offender (no = 0; yes = 1 [*O negotiated*])
	OREASSUR	Offender reassured the victim (no = 0; yes = 1 [*O reassured*])
	OTAKESOU	Offender took souvenirs from victim (no = 0; yes = 1 [*Took souveni*])
	OTAKEOTH	Offender took other items (no = 0; yes = 1 [*Took oth item*])
	WHOREMCL	Who removed victim's clothing (not or self-removed = 0; O disrobed V = 1 [*O disrobed V*])
	CLOTHCAR	Clothes were removed carefully (else = 0; yes [2] = 1 [*Care clothin*])
	CLOTHDAM	Clothes were damaged when removed (else = 0; yes [3, 4] = 1 [*Damagd cloth*])
	OREDRESV	Victim redressed by offender (no = 0; yes = 1 [*Redressed V*])
	OAVDETEC	Offender took steps to avoid detection (no = 0; yes = 1 [*O avd detect*])
	OCOVIDEN	Offender covered up identity (no = 0; yes = 1 [*O hid ident*])
	OWEAPINV	Evidence offender used a weapon (no = 0; yes = 1] [*Used weapon*])
	WEAPLOC	Location of weapons used (found = 0; brought/ brought and found = 1 [*Weapon broug*])
	OWEAPREM	Offender removed weapon from scene (no = 0; yes = 1 [*Removed weap*])

(*continued on next page*)

Variable group	Variable label	Definition (category labels and coding; numbers in parentheses indicated categories combined in the code)
	WEAPREC	Weapon was recovered (no = 0; yes = 1 [*Weapon recov*])
	STABBING	Offender used stabbing/cutting weapon (no = 0; yes = 1 [*Used knife*])
	OTHRWEAP	Offender used other type of weapon (no = 0; yes = 1 [*Used oth weap*])
	OFETISH	Offender displayed obvious fetish (no = 0; yes = 1 [*Fetish beh*])
	OTORTURE	Offender tortured victim (no = 0; yes = 1 [*Tortured V*])
	USERESTR	Offender used restraints on victim (no = 0; yes = 1 [*Used binding*])
	OGAGGEDV	Offender gagged the victim (no = 0; yes = 1 [*Gagged V*])
	BLNDFLDV	Offender blindfolded victim (no = 0; yes = 1 [*Blindfold V*])
	VFACECOV	Offender covered victim's face (no = 0; yes = 1 [*V face cover*])
	WEAPWOUN	Victim was stabbed or shot (no = 0; yes = 1 [*V stab/shot*])
	BEATING	Victim showed blunt force injuries (no = 0; yes = 1 [*V beaten*])
	AIRWAY	Victim trauma involved airway or breathing (no = 0; yes = 1 [*Strang/drown*])
	BLUNTTRA	Victim showed evidence of blunt trauma (no = 0; yes = 1 [*Blunt trauma*])
	FACETRAU	Victim suffered blunt force trauma to the face (no = 0; yes = 1 [*Face trauma*])
	OBITEV	Offender bit victim (no = 0; yes = 1 [*O bit V*])

Italic text indicates multidimensional scaling coordinate label for Figs. 7.1–7.4.

Appendix C

Property Vectors

Serial Rape CAP Model (Chapter 7)

From: *Criminal Profiling: Principles and Practice*
By: R. N. Kocsis © Humana Press Inc., Totowa, NJ

Table 1

Summaries of the Composition of Victim Characteristic Clusters Used in the Property Vector MDS Fitting Analyses

Victim Characteristics Variable Set

Average β Weight Dimension 1	Average β Weight Dimension 2	Canonical Correlation	Individual β Weight Dimension 1	Individual β Weight Dimension 2	Regression Multiple R	Cluster Identifier	Variable	Hierarchical Clustering using Ward's method
			.181	-.739	.74		VLIVEWTH	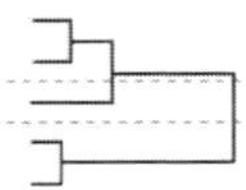
.386	-.613	.75	.591	-.488	.71	VICTIM 1	VTRANSPT	
.632	.222	.70	.632	.222	.70	VICTIM 2	VINCAPAC	
			-.379	.212	.41		VSEX	
-.462	.383	..68	-.544	.554	.72	VICTIM 3	VAGE	

Each variable included in this table achieved a significant ($p < 0.05$) multiple r value when predicted by the two-dimensional coordinates from the multidimensional scaling (MDS) solution.

Table 2
Summaries of the Composition of Offender Characteristic Clusters Used in the Property Vector MDS Fitting Analyses

Offender Characteristics Variable Set

			.121	.859	.89		OLANG
.051	.869	.93	.044	.868	.87	OFFENDER 1	OEYECOL
			-.013	.879	.88		ORACE
			-.208	.570	.57		OACCENT
			-.233	.565	.55		OINTERNA
-.363	.490	.79	-.259	.546	.56	OFFENDER 2	OFACHAIR
			-.422	.499	.59		OHAIRCOL
			-.456	.388	.54		OHAIRSHA
			-.599	.372	.64		OODOURS
			-.482	.091	.47		OCONFESS
-.531	.011	.60	-.579	-.069	.59	OFFENDER 3	OVEHTYPE
			-.496	-.494	.79		OHEIGHT
-.066	-.528	.91	-.162	-.748	.80	OFFENDER 4	OPOSPROP
			.087	-.374	.37		OLIFESTY
			.306	-.497	.55		OVEHUSED
			.584	.036	.59		OSCAR
.511	.132	.79	.560	.201	.63	OFFENDER 5	OBUILD
			.468	.150	.52		ODRUGALC
			.431	.142	.47		OWEIGHT
			.464	.329	.62		OCRIMST
			.345	.296	.50		OOUTFEAT
.273	.356	.82	.351	.500	.67	OFFENDER 6	OMENTILL
			.112	.413	.45		OMARITAL
			.179	.337	.412		OLIVEWTH
			.185	.260	.347		OAGE

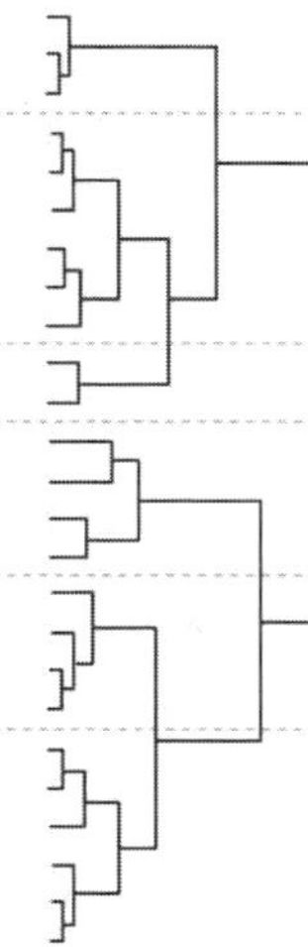

Each variable included in this table achieved a significant ($p < 0.05$) multiple r value when predicted by the two-dimensional coordinates from the multidimensional scaling (MDS) solution.

Table 3
Summaries of the Composition of Offender–Victim Interaction Characteristic Clusters Used in the Property Vector MDS Fitting Analyses

Offender–Victim Interaction Characteristics Variable Set

Average β Weight Dimension 1	Average β Weight Dimension 2	Canonical Correlation	Individual β Weight Dimension 1	Individual β Weight Dimension 2	Regression Multiple R	Cluster Identifier	Variable	Hierarchical Clustering using Ward's method
.410	-.420	.85	.357	-.383	.47	INTERACT 1	CFINCONT	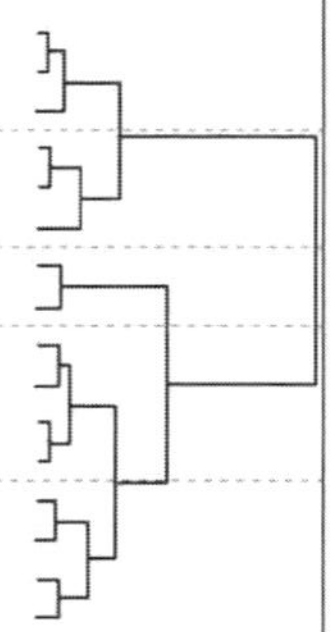
			.354	-.416	.49		IPOTWITN	
			.518	-.461	.59		CLIVQUAR	
.639	-.027	.74	.746	-.208	.73	INTERACT 2	IOUTDOOR	
			.735	-.102	.72		ICONTACT	
			.437	.229	.53		INEIGHBR	
-.038	.511	.72	.086	.432	.46	INTERACT 3	CPUBPLAC	
			-.163	.590	.59		RCSAME	
-.568	.357	.80	-.431	.254	.46	INTERACT 4	IVCLOTH	
			-.524	.506	.62		CINOUT	
			-.659	.356	.69		CISAME	
			-.657	.311	.67		RISAME	
-.635	-.033	.83	-.602	.147	.58	INTERACT 5	COUTDOOR	
			-.678	.064	.67		ILIVQUAR	
			-.533	-.137	.59		CFAMSITE	
			-.727	-.206	.79		IFAMSITE	

Each variable included in this table achieved a significant ($p < 0.05$) multiple r value when predicted by the two-dimensional coordinates from the multidimensional scaling (MDS) solution.

Appendix D

Labels and Definitions for All Variables in Chapter 8

Sexual Murder CAP Model

Variable group	Variable label	Definition (category labels and coding; numbers in parentheses indicated categories combined in the code)
Victim characteristics	VSEX	Victim's sex (male = 0; female = 1)
	VRACE	Victim's race (white = 0; non-white = 1)
	VAGE	Victim's age (20 yrs old or less = 0; 21 years or older = 1)
	VHEIGHT	Victim's height (short = 0; medium, tall = 1)
	VBUILD	Victim's build (small = 0; medium, large = 1)
	VHAIRLEN	Victim's hair length (short/none [1–3] = 0; medium/long [4–6] = 1)
	VGLASSES	Victim wears glasses/sunglasses (no = 0; yes = 1)
	VSCARS	Victim had scars/marks (no = 0; yes = 1)
	VOUTFEAT	Victim had outstanding physical features (no = 0; yes = 1)
	VTRANSPT	Victim's usual mode of transport (self-modes [1, 2, 4] = 0; relies on others [3, 5, 6, 7] = 1)
	VMARITAL	Victim's marital status (single/ex-partner [1, 3, 4, 5, 6] = 0; partnered [2] = 1)
	VLIVEWTH	Victim living with (alone [8] = 0; others [1–7] = 1)
	VLIFESTY	Victim's general lifestyle (non-criminal [1, 2, 4, 8, 11–13] = 0; criminal [3, 5–7, 9–10] = 1)

(*continued on next page*)

Variable group	Variable label	Definition (category labels and coding; numbers in parentheses indicated categories combined in the code)
	VINCAPAC	Victim incapacitated at time of initial contact (no = 0; yes = 1)
Offender characteristics	ORACE	Offender's race (white = 0; non-white = 1)
	OAGE	Offender's age (20 yrs old or less = 0; 21 years or older = 1)
	OLANG	Offender's language background (monolingual = 0; bilingual = 1)
	OHEIGHT	Offender's height (short = 0; medium, tall = 1)
	OBUILD	Offender's build (small = 0; medium, large = 1)
	OHAIRLEN	Offender's hair length (short/none [1–3] =0; medium/long [4–6] =1)
	OHAIRSTY	Offender's hair style (neat/tidy = 0; unkempt = 1)
	OGLASSES	Offender wears glasses (no = 0; yes = 1)
	OFACHAIR	Offender had facial hair (no = 0; yes = 1)
	OSCAR	Offender had scars/marks (no = 0; yes = 1)
	OOUTFEAT	Offender had outstanding physical features (no = 0; yes = 1)
	OGROOM	Offender appeared well-groomed (no = 0; yes = 1)
	OACCENT	Offender had an accent (no = 0; yes = 1)
	OMENTILL	Offender showed evidence of mental illness (no = 0; yes = 1)
	ODRUGALC	Offender showed evidence of drug/alcohol use (no = 0; yes = 1)
	OUNUSUAL	Offender showed unusual characteristics (no = 0; yes = 1)
	OINTERST	Offender visited interstate in past 10 years (no = 0; yes = 1)
	OINTERNA	Offender lived/visited internationally over past 10 years (no = 0; yes = 1)
	OMARITAL	Offender's marital status (single/ex-partner [1, 3, 4, 5] = 0; partnered [2] = 1)
	OLIVEWTH	Offender living with (alone [8] = 0; others [1–7] = 1)
	OJOBTYPE	Offender job type (unemployed = 0; employed = 1)
	OLIFESTY	Offender's general lifestyle (non-criminal [1, 2, 4, 8, 11–13] = 0; criminal [3, 5–7, 9–10] = 1)
	OTRANSPT	Offender's usual mode of transport (self- modes [1, 2, 4] = 0; relies on others [3, 5, 6, 7] = 1)
	OCRIMST	Offender's criminal status (non-offender = 0; statutory release = 1)

(*continued on next page*)

Variable group	Variable label	Definition (category labels and coding; numbers in parentheses indicated categories combined in the code)
	OPRSEXOF	Offender had prior sex offences (no = 0; yes = 1)
	OSEXHAB	Offender's sexual habits (heterosexual = 0; homosexual/bisexual = 1)
	OPORNCOL	Offender had a collection of pornography (no = 0; yes = 1)
	ODETCOLL	Offender had a collection of detective magazines (no = 0; yes = 1)
	OSEXPARA	Offender had a collection of sexual paraphernalia (no = 0; yes = 1)
	OMENPROB	Offender displayed symptoms or had been treated for mental problems (no = 0; yes = 1)
	OCONFESS	Offender admitted to other similar crimes of violence (no = 0; yes = 1)
	OVEHUSED	Offender used a vehicle in this incident (no = 0; yes = 1)
	OVEHSTAT	Offender's vehicle status (owned = 0; not owned = 1)
	OVEHTYPE	Offender's vehicle type (car = 0; van/SUV/truck = 1)
	OVEHCOND	Offender's vehicle condition (less than immaculate [2, 3, 4] = 0; exceptionally good [1] = 1)
	OVEHAGE	Offender's vehicle age (newer = 0; older [2, 3] = 1)
Offender–victim interaction characteristics	IPRIORAC	Prior activity initial contact area (no = 0; yes = 1)
	IPOTWITN	Potential witnesses at initial contact area (no = 0; yes = 1)
	ICONTACT	Location of initial contact scene (indoors = 0; outdoors = 1)
	ICOMMUN	Community type for initial contact scene (city [2, 3] = 0; non-city [1, 4, 5] = 1)
	ILIVQUAR	Initial contact: living quarters (no = 0; yes = 1)
	IPUBPLAC	Initial contact: public place (no = 0; yes = 1)
	IOUTDOOR	Initial contact: outdoors (no = 0; yes = 1)
	IFAMSITE	Offender's familiarity with initial contact site (familiar = 0; unfamiliar = 1)
	IVCLOTH	Victim's clothing at initial contact site (nothing done [1] = 0; something done [2–5] = 1)
	CISAME	Initial contact site same as crime site (no = 0; yes = 1)
	CINOUT	Crime site was indoors or outdoors (indoors = 0; outdoors = 1)

(*continued on next page*)

Variable group	Variable label	Definition (category labels and coding; numbers in parentheses indicated categories combined in the code)
	CCOMMUM	Crime scene community type (city [2, 3] = 0; non-city [1, 4, 5] = 1)
	CLIVQUAR	Crime scene: living quarters (no = 0; yes = 1)
	CPUBPLAC	Crime scene: public place (no = 0; yes = 1)
	COUTDOOR	Crime scene: outdoors (no = 0; yes = 1)
	CFAMSITE	Offender's familiarity with crime scene (familiar = 0; unfamiliar = 1)
	CVCLOTH	Victim's clothing at crime scene (nothing done (1) = 0; something done (2-5) = 1)
	RISAME	Recovery site same as initial contact site (no = 0; yes = 1)
	RCSAME	Recovery site same as crime scene (no = 0; yes = 1)
	RCOMMUN	Recovery site community type (city [2, 3] = 0; non-city [1, 4, 5] = 1)
	RFAMSITE	Offender's familiarity with recovery site (familiar = 0; unfamiliar = 1)
	RVCLOTH	Victim's clothing at recovery site (nothing done [1] = 0; something done [2–5] = 1)
Crime scene characteristics	RMOVEVIC	Offender moved victim's body from crime to recovery site (no = 0; yes = 1 [*Body moved*])
	DISPOPEN	Victim's body was openly displayed (no = 0; yes = 1 [*No hide body*])
	DISPHID	Victim's body was hidden (no = 0; yes = 1 [*Hid body*])
	DISPLACK	Apparent lack of concern over body display (no = 0; yes = 1 [*No care body*])
	RCLOTHMV	Clothing on victim (fully clothed = 0; Clothing removed or shifted = 1 [*Cloth distur*])
	POSPRONE	Position of body was prone (no = 0; yes = 1 [*Body prone*])
	POSSUPIN	Position of body was supine (no = 0; yes = 1 [*Body supine*])
	POSOTHER	Position of body was found not lying down (3-6) (no = 0; yes = 1 [*Body other*])
	OVRELAT	Offender's relationship to victim (stranger = 0; acquaintance = 1 [*O acquaint V*])
	OVSELEC	Offender's selection of the victim (opportunistic = 0; planned = 1 [*Plan attack*])

(*continued on next page*)

Variable group	Variable label	Definition (category labels and coding; numbers in parentheses indicated categories combined in the code)
	FORCEBEF	Force was used before sex (no = 0; yes = 1 [*Force bf sex*])
	FORCEDUR	Force was used during sex (no = 0; yes = 1 [*Force dg sex*])
	FORCEAFT	Force was used after sex (no = 0; yes = 1 [*Force af sex*])
	FORCERES	Force was used when victim resisted (no = 0; yes = 1 [*Force resist*])
	OANGER	Extent of offender anger evident (none/some = 0; extreme = 1 [*Anger extrem*])
	VICRESIS	Victim offered resistance (no resistance = 0; some resistance = 1 [*V resisted*])
	REACTRES	Reaction to victim resistance (ignore/back down = 0; threaten/force = 1 [*O threaten*])
	SEXACTV	Evidence of sex act with victim (no = 0; yes = 1 [*Sex with V*])
	SEXASSAU	Nature of sexual assault (assaulted internally = 0; assaulted externally = 1 [*External sex*])
	SEMENBOD	Semen found in body cavities of victim (no = 0; yes = 1 [*Semen in bod*])
	SEMENOTH	Semen found elsewhere (no = 0; yes = 1 [*Semen elsewh*])
	PMORTSEX	Postmortem sex act evident (no = 0; yes = 1 [*Postmort sex*])
	OSEXDUSF	Evidence of offender sex dysfunction (no = 0; yes = 1 [*O sex dysfun*])
	NONPENIS	Objects other than penis inserted into victim (no = 0; yes = 1 [*Object inser*])
	OATTCHG	Evidence of change in offender attitude toward victim (no = 0; yes = 1 [*O chgd att V*])
	OIMAGEV	Offender image projected to victim (neutral = 0; managed [1, 3] = 1 [*O manip imag*])
	ODEMEANV	Offender demeanor to victim (neutral = 0; managed [1, 3] = 1 [*O manip beh*])
	VONEGOT	Negotiation between victim and offender (no = 0; yes = 1 [*O negotiated*])
	OREASSUR	Offender reassured the victim (no = 0; yes = 1 [*O reassured*])
	OCOMCRIM	Offender communicated about crime to others (no = 0; yes = 1 [*O Comm Crime*])

(*continued on next page*)

Variable group	Variable label	Definition (category labels and coding; numbers in parentheses indicated categories combined in the code)
	OTAKESOU	Offender took souvenirs from victim (no = 0; yes = 1 [*Took souveni*])
	OTAKEOTH	Offender took other items (no = 0; yes = 1 [*Took oth item*])
	WHOREMCL	Who removed victim's clothing (not or self-removed = 0; O disrobed V = 1 [*O disrobed V*])
	CLOTHCAR	Clothes were removed carefully (else = 0; yes [2] = 1 [*Care clothin*])
	CLOTHDAM	Clothes were damaged when removed (else = 0; yes [3, 4] = 1 [*Damagd cloth*])
	OREDRESV	Victim redressed by offender (no = 0; yes = 1 [*Redressed V*])
	OPRECAUT	Offender took precautions to avoid apprehension (no = 0; yes = 1 [*Took precaut*])
	OWEAPINV	Evidence offender used a weapon (no = 0; yes = 1 [*Used weapon*])
	WEAPLOC	Location of weapons used (found = 0; brought/brought and found = 1) [*Weapon broug*])
	OWEAPREM	Offender removed weapon from scene (no = 0; yes = 1 [*Removed weap*])
	LIGATURE	Offender used ligature weapon (no = 0; yes = 1 [*Used ligatur*])
	BLUDGEON	Offender used bludgeoning weapon (no = 0; yes = 1 [*Used bludgeo*])
	STABBING	Offender used stabbing weapon (no = 0; yes = 1 [*Used knife*])
	FIREARM	Offender used firearm (no = 0; yes = 1 [*Used firearm*])
	OPROPUSE	Offender used special props (no = 0; yes = 1 [*Used props*])
	OFETISH	Offender displayed obvious fetish (no = 0; yes = 1 [*Fetish beh*])
	OTORTURE	Offender tortured victim (no = 0; yes = 1 [*Tortured V*])
	USERESTR	Offender used restraints on victim (no = 0; yes = 1 [*Used binding*])
	RESTRLOC	Location of restraints used (found = 0; brought/brought and found = 1 [*Binding broug*])
	OREMREST	Offender removed restraints from scene (no = 0; yes = 1 [*Binding remov*])

(*continued on next page*)

Variable group	Variable label	Definition (category labels and coding; numbers in parentheses indicated categories combined in the code)
	RESTNEAT	Offender removed restraints from scene (no = 0; yes = 1 [*Binding remov*])
	OGAGGEDV	Offender gagged the victim (no = 0; yes = 1 [*Gagged V*])
	AIRWAY	Victim trauma involved airway or breathing (no = 0; yes = 1 [*Strang/drown*])
	BEATING	Victim showed blunt force injuries (no = 0; yes = 1 [*V beaten*])
	BURNING	Victim was burned (no = 0; yes = 1 [*V burned*])
	WEAPWOUN	Victim was stabbed or shot (no = 0; yes = 1 [*V stab/shot*])
	SINGTRLO	Victim trauma isolated to a single body location (no = 0; yes = 1 [*Singl trauma*])
	MULTTRLO	Victim trauma observed at multiple body locations (no = 0; yes = 1 [*Mulpl trauma*])
	MINORTRA	Victim suffered minor blunt force trauma (no = 0; yes = 1 [*Minor trauma*])
	MAJORTRA	Victim suffered major blunt force trauma (no = 0; yes = 1 [*Major trauma*])
	FACETRAU	Victim suffered blunt force trauma to the face (no = 0; yes = 1 [*Facial traum*])
	OTHFACIA	Victim suffered other facial injuries (no = 0; yes = 1 [*Other facial*])
	VDISMEMB	Victim was dismembered (no = 0; yes = 1 [*Dismember V*])
	UNPATTER	Victims wounds were generally unpatterned (no = 0; yes [all but 7, 12] = 1) [*Unpatt wound*])
	PATTERND	Victims wounds were generally patterned (no = 0; yes [7, 12] = 1 [*Pattern wound*])

Italic text indicates multidimensional scaling coordinate label for Figs. 8.1–8.4.

Appendix E

Property Vectors

Sexual Murder CAP Model (Chapter 8)

From: *Criminal Profiling: Principles and Practice*
By: R. N. Kocsis © Humana Press Inc., Totowa, NJ

Table 1
Summaries of the Composition of Victim Characteristic Clusters Used in the Property Vector MDS Fitting Analyses

Victim Characteristics Variable Set								
Average β Weight Dimension 1	Average β Weight Dimension 2	Canonical Correlation	Individual β Weight Dimension 1	Individual β Weight Dimension 2	Regression Multiple R	Cluster Identifier	Variable	Hierarchical Clustering using Ward's method
			-.536	.324	.61		VGLASSES	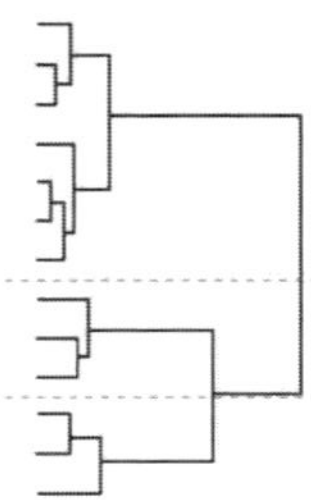
			-.467	.411	.60		VSCARS	
			-.385	.395	.53		VOUTFEAT	
-.334	.416	.80	-.236	.324	.39	VICTIM 1	VAGE	
			-.266	.433	.49		VBUILD	
			-.257	.478	.53		VSEX	
			-.190	.550	.57		VHAIRLEN	
			.339	.277	.44		VHEIGHT	
.364	.118	.61	.546	.067	.53	VICTIM 2	VLIFESTY	
			.234	-.052	.24		VTRANSPT	
			.136	-.527	.54		VRACE	
-.292	-.467	.81	-.160	-.355	.39	VICTIM 3	VLIVEWTH	
			-.671	-.395	.78		VINCAPAC	

Each variable included in this table achieved a significant ($p < 0.05$) multiple r value when predicted by the two-dimensional coordinates from the multidimensional scaling (MDS) solution.

Table 2

Summaries of the Composition of Offender Characteristic Clusters Used in the Property Vector MDS Fitting Analyses

Offender Characteristics Variable Set								
Average β Weight Dimension 1	Average β Weight Dimension 2	Canonical Correlation	Individual β Weight Dimension 1	Individual β Weight Dimension 2	Regression Multiple R	Cluster Identifier	Variable	Hierarchical Clustering using Ward's method
-.269	.362	.89	-.453	.448	.33	OFFENDER 1	OACCENT	
			-.612	.271	.34		OINTERNA	
			.052	.325	.42		OLIVEWTH	
			.019	.335	.63		OHAIRLEN	
			-.116	.405	.59		OVEHSTAT	
			-.445	.402	.66		OSCAR	
-.334	-.160	.69	-.460	-.101	.53	OFFENDER 2	OHAIRSTY	
			-.222	-.346	.42		OTRANSPT	
			-.527	-.054	.47		ORACE	
			.124	-.470	.41		OHEIGHT	
			-.391	-.159	.49		OMENTILL	
.412	-.422	.93	.346	-.386	.75	OFFENDER 3	OSEXHAB	
			.707	-.276	.74		OJOBTYPE	
			.547	-.542	.50		ODRUGALC	
			.268	-.467	.55		OVEHAGE	
			.222	-.446	.52		OPORNCOL	
			.381	-.415	.49		OVEHCOND	
.395	.198	.88	.374	.339	.37	OFFENDER 4	OGROOM	
			.351	-.109	.46		OVEHTYPE	
			.220	.554	.25		ODETCOLL	
			.219	.129	.59		OMARITAL	
			.403	.204	.45		OMENPROB	
			.609	.477	.50		OLANG	
			.462	-.011	.77		OVEHUSED	
.678	-.029	.91	.726	-.081	.72	OFFENDER 5	OCRIMST	
			.613	.011	.61		OINTERST	
			.711	.102	.63		OPRSEXOF	
			.625	-.029	.73		OAGE	
			.822	-.040	.82		OSEXPARA	

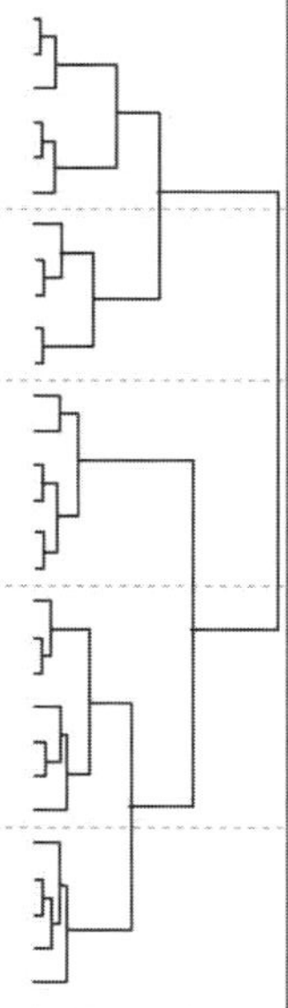

Each variable included in this table achieved a significant ($p < 0.05$) multiple r value when predicted by the two-dimensional coordinates from the multidimensional scaling (MDS) solution.

Table 3
Summaries of the Composition of Offender–Victim Interaction Characteristic Clusters Used in the Property Vector MDS Fitting Analyses

Offender–Victim Interaction Characteristics Variable Set								
Average β Weight Dimension 1	**Average β Weight Dimension 2**	**Canonical Correlation**	**Individual β Weight Dimension 1**	**Individual β Weight Dimension 2**	**Regression Multiple R**	**Cluster Identifier**	**Variable**	**Hierarchical Clustering using Ward's method**
-.305	-.359	.81	-.445	-.487	.66	INTERACT 1	ILIVQUAR	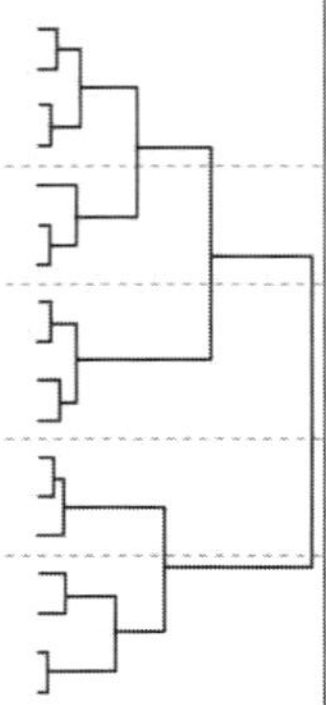
			-.181	-.419	.45		CPUBPLAC	
			-.274	-.272	.38		IPRIORAC	
			-.202	-.239	.31		IPUBPLAC	
-.753	-.052	.81	-.578	-.330	.66	INTERACT 2	CISAME	
			-.619	-.096	.63		RISAME	
			-.738	.066	.74		IVCLOTH	
-.331	.353	.64	-.323	.395	.51	INTERACT 3	COUTDOOR	
			-.305	.303	.43		CINOUT	
			-.267	.126	.30		RCSAME	
			-.175	.326	.37		CFAMSITE	
.524	.439	.85	.517	.514	.75	INTERACT 4	IOUTDOOR	
			.468	.423	.65		RVCLOTH	
			.588	.380	.72		ICONTACT	
.556	-.125	.76	.695	.134	.72	INTERACT 5	ICOMMUN	
			.511	.019	.51		CVCLOTH	
			.522	-.288	.58		CLIVQUAR	
			.537	-.334	.61		RCOMMUN	

Each variable included in this table achieved a significant ($p < 0.05$) multiple r value when predicted by the two-dimensional coordinates from the multidimensional scaling (MDS) solution.

Appendix F

Labels and Definitions for All Variables in Chapter 9

Serial Arson CAP Model

Variable set	Variable label	Definition (category labels and coding)
Personal offender characteristics	OAGE	Offender's age (20 years old or less = 0; 21 years or older = 1)
	OLANG	Offender's language background (monolingual = 0; bilingual = 1)
	OBUILD	Offender's build (small = 0; medium, large = 1)
	OHAIRSHA	Offender's hair shade (lighter = 0; darker = 1)
	OHAIRLEN	Offender's hair length (short/none [1–3] = 0; medium/long [4–6] = 1)
	OHAIRCOL	Offender's hair color (red, gray, or white = 0; brown or black = 1)
	OEYECOL	Offender's eye color (light eyes = 0; dark eyes = 1)
	OTEETH	Offender's teeth (not noticed = 0; noticeably imperfect = 1)
	OFACHAIR	Offender had facial hair (no = 0; yes = 1)
	OOUTFEAT	Offender had outstanding physical features (no = 0; yes = 1)
	OACCENT	Offender had an accent (no = 0; yes = 1)
	OODOUR	Offender had noticeable odor (no = 0; yes = 1)
General offender behavior variables	ODRUGALC	Offender showed evidence of drug/alcohol use (no = 0; yes = 1)
	OINTERST	Offender visited interstate in past 10 years (no = 0; yes = 1)

(*continued on next page*)

Variable set	Variable label	Definition (category labels and coding)
	OINTERNA	Offender lived/visited internationally over past 10 years (no = 0; yes = 1)
	OLIVEWTH	Offender living with (alone [8] = 0; others [1–7] = 1)
	OJOBTYPE	Offender job type (unemployed = 0; employed = 1)
	OLIFESTY	Offender's general lifestyle (non-criminal [1, 2, 4, 8, 11–13] = 0; criminal [3, 5–7, 9–10] = 1)
	OCRIMST	Offender's criminal status (non-offender = 0; statutory release = 1)
	OSEXHAB	Offender's sexual habits (heterosexual = 0; homosexual/bisexual = 1)
	OMENPROB	Offender displayed symptoms or had been treated for mental problems (no = 0; yes = 1)
	OPOSPROP	Offender possessed other's property (no = 0; yes = 1)
	OCONFESS	Offender admitted to other similar crimes of violence (no = 0; yes = 1)
	OVEHUSED	Offender used a vehicle in this incident (no = 0; yes = 1)
	OVEHSTAT	Offender's vehicle status (owned = 0; not owned = 1)
	OVEHTYPE	Offender's vehicle type (car = 0; van/SUV/truck = 1)
Event-specific offender behavior and choices variables	THREAT	Offender makes a threat to someone about committing the arson (no = 0; yes = 1)
	DISTMAJ	Offender travels more than 1 km to the target (no = 0; yes = 1)
	DISTMIN	Offender travels less than 1 km to the target (no = 0; yes = 1)
	ACCOMPLI	Offender had accomplices in committing the arson (no = 0; yes = 1)
	VISIBLE	Offender lit fire in highly visible location with potential witnesses (no = 0; yes = 1)
	PRESENT	Offender was present at the crime scene watching the fire (no = 0; yes = 1)
	NOTPRES	Offender was not present at the crime scene watching the fire (no = 0; yes = 1)
	ACALLS	Offender reports the fire he actually started himself (no = 0; yes = 1)
	AEXTIN	Offender is involved in attempts to extinguish the fire he actually set (no = 0; yes = 1)
	NIGHT	Offender set the fire at night (no = 0; yes = 1)

(*continued on next page*)

Variable set	Variable label	Definition (category labels and coding)
	DAY	Offender set the fire during the day (no = 0; yes = 1)
	WEEK	Offender set the fire on a weekday (no = 0; yes = 1)
	WEEKEND	Offender set the fire on a weekend day (no = 0; yes = 1)
	HOLIDAY	Offender set the fire during some type of holiday period (no = 0; yes = 1)
	SUMSPRIG	Offender set the fire during the summer or spring—warm season (no = 0; yes = 1)
	WINAUTM	Offender set the fire during the winter or autumn—cold season (no = 0; yes = 1)
Crime scene variables	SINGPOO	Fire was lit from a single point of origin or location (no = 0; yes = 1)
	MULTIPOO	Fire was lit from multiple points of origin or locations (no = 0; yes = 1)
	POOEXTER	Point of origin of fire was a location exterior to the target (no = 0; yes = 1)
	POOINT	Point of origin of fire was a location interior to the target (no = 0; yes = 1)
	MATERBRO	Offender consciously brought materials to start the fire with him to the target (no = 0; yes = 1)
	ACCELERA	An accelerant was employed by the offender to light the fire (no = 0; yes = 1)
	TRAILERS	There was evidence of a trailer (detectable burn line of liquid accelerant) used at the fire (no = 0; yes = 1)
	PLANNED	There was evidence the arson was planned with a specific intended target (no = 0; yes = 1)
	RANDOM	There was evidence that the arson was unplanned or random (no = 0; yes = 1)
	ENTARGET	Offender actually entered the target to light the fire (no = 0; yes = 1)
	MAJFIRE	The resulting fire caused major damage (no = 0; yes = 1)
	MINFIRE	The resulting fire caused minor damage (no = 0; yes = 1)
	SPECBURN	Specific items were initially burned by the offender to start the fire (no = 0; yes = 1)
	ADAMAGE	Additional damage, other than fire damage, was caused by the offender (e.g., vandalism) (no = 0; yes = 1)

(*continued on next page*)

Variable set	Variable label	Definition (category labels and coding)
	THEFT	Offender stole something from the target (no = 0; yes = 1)
	EVIDENCE	Physical evidence was left by the offender at the crime scene (no = 0; yes = 1)
	SEXACTIV	There was evidence that the offender engaged in some sexual activity at the crime scene (no = 0; yes = 1)
	RESPROP	The target was a residential property such as a house or apartment (no = 0; yes = 1)
	COMPROP	The target was a commercial property such as a business, used for work, not living (no = 0; yes = 1)
	EDUPROP	The target was an educational facility such as a school (no = 0; yes = 1)
	STATPROP	The target was a state-owned property such as a government building or police station (no = 0; yes = 1)
	VEHPROP	The target was a motor vehicle such as a car, motorcycle, or truck (no = 0; yes = 1)
	MINPROP	The target was a minor item such as a rubbish b in, letter box or abandoned property (no = 0; yes = 1)
	BUSPROP	The target was a bushland or forest, possibly including property fences and hedges (no = 0; yes = 1)
	TOCCUPY	The target was occupied by people at the time of the fire (no = 0; yes = 1)
	TUNOCCUP	The target was not occupied by people at the time of the fire (no = 0; yes = 1)
	TRELATIO	The offender had some relationship with the target such as their school or workplace (no = 0; yes = 1)
	TUNRELAT	The offender had no relationship with the target
	TSECURTY	The target had some form of security system, fire alarm, sprinkler systems, and so on (no = 0; yes = 1)

Appendix G

Fit Statistics for External Offender-Related Property Vectors

Serial Arson CAP Model (Chapter 9)

From: *Criminal Profiling: Principles and Practice*
By: R. N. Kocsis © Humana Press Inc., Totowa, NJ

Variable	β Weight for dimension 1	β Weight for dimension 2	Multiple correlation	Omnibus F-test	p Value
Personal set					
Significant variables[a]					
OLANG	–0.57	–0.09	0.58	6.54	0.01
OHAIRCOL	0.31	0.46	0.57	6.04	0.01
OEYECOL	0.54	0.19	0.58	6.41	0.01
OTEETH	0.38	–0.33	0.49	3.92	0.03
OUTFEAT	0.33	–0.37	0.49	3.92	0.03
OACCENT	–0.66	0.16	0.67	10.44	<0.01
Nonsignificant variables					
OAGE, OBUILD, OHAIRSHA, OHAIRLEN, OFACHAIR, OODOUR					
General set					
Significant variables					
OINTERST	0.22	0.63	0.66	9.43	<0.01
OINTERNA	–0.73	0.18	0.75	15.49	<0.01
OLIVEWTH	0.33	–0.70	0.78	18.75	<0.01
OJOBTYPE	0.24	–0.48	0.54	4.91	0.02
ODRGALCO	0.43	–0.25	0.52	4.53	0.02
OCRIMSTA	–0.36	0.40	0.57	5.76	0.01
OCONFESS	–0.33	–0.35	0.46	3.31	0.05
OVEHUSED	–0.51	0.43	0.67	10.45	<0.01
OVEHSTAT	0.67	0.10	0.68	10.95	<0.01
Nonsignificant	variables				
OLIFESTY, OSEXHAB, OMENPROB, OPOSPROP, OVEHTYPE					
Event-specific set					
Significant variables					
DISTMAJ	–0.48	–0.56	0.74	15.20	<0.01

DISTMIN	0.48	0.56	0.74	15.20	<0.01
ACCOMPLI	0.16	–0.65	0.67	10.75	<0.01
VISIBLE	0.19	–0.62	0.65	9.52	<0.01
PRESENT	0.52	0.07	0.53	4.99	0.01
NOTPRES	–0.52	–0.07	0.53	4.99	0.01
WEEK	0.40	0.72	0.69	9.35	<0.01
WEEKEND	–0.40	–0.72	0.69	9.35	<0.01
HOLIDAY	–0.28	0.37	0.54	4.29	0.03
SUMSPRIG	–0.48	–0.54	0.58	5.31	0.01
WINAUTM	0.48	0.54	0.58	5.31	0.01
Nonsignificant variables					
THREAT, ACALLS, AEXTIN, NIGHT, DAY					
Offender set					
OFF_1	0.22	–0.45	0.50	4.31	0.02
OFF_2	–0.50	–0.06	0.50	4.35	0.02
OFF_3 (not significantly predicted)	0.32	–0.29	0.43	3.05	0.07
OFF_4	0.12	–0.50	0.51	4.56	0.02
OFF_5	0.14	–0.58	0.59	7.08	<0.01
OFF_6 (not significantly predicted)	<–0.01	0.01	0.01	<0.01	1.0
OFF_7	0.14	–0.47	0.49	4.16	0.03
OFF_8	0.14	–0.47	0.49	4.16	0.03
OFF_9	0.14	–0.47	0.49	4.16	0.03
OFF_10 (not significantly predicted)	0.21	0.17	0.27	1.05	0.37
OFF_11 (not significantly predicted)	0.1	–0.43	0.43	2.95	0.07
OFF_12 (not significantly predicted)	0.18	–0.25	0.30	1.31	0.29
OFF_13 (not significantly predicted)	0.40	<0.01	0.40	2.45	0.11

[a]Only significant offender-related variables will have the fitted property vectors displayed in Figures 2 through 5.

Index